CHANGING THE
Public Health

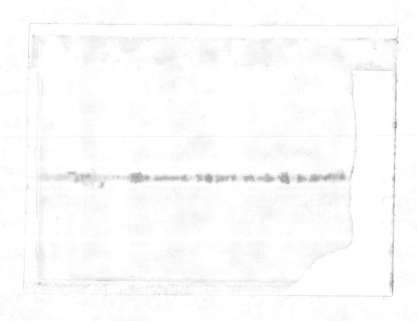

CHANGING THE
Public Health

Research Unit in Health and Behavioural Change
University of Edinburgh

JOHN WILEY & SONS
Chichester · New York · Brisbane · Toronto · Singapore

Library of Congress Cataloging-in-Publication Data

Changing the public health.

Bibliography: p.
Includes index.
1. Health behavior. 2. Social medicine. 3. Health promotion. 4. Health education. I. University of Edinburgh. Research Unit in Health and Behavioural Change. [DNLM: 1. Attitude to Health. 2. Health Education. 3. Health Promotion. 4. Public Health. 5. Social Change. WA 30 C456]
RA776.9.C48   1989.   362.1   88-5610
ISBN 0 471 91976 4 (pbk.)

British Library Cataloguing in Publication Data

Changing the public health.
1. Public health.
I. University of Edinburgh, Research Unit in Health and Behavioural Change
614

ISBN 0 471 91976 4

Phototypeset by Input Typesetting Ltd, London
Printed in Great Britain by Dotesios Ltd, Trowbridge, Wiltshire

FOR ROGAN

Contents

Contributors

This book was written collaboratively by members of the core staff of the Research Unit in Health and Behavioural Change at the University of Edinburgh.

Kathryn Backett MA PhD Research Fellow; *formerly Research Fellow in the Department of Sociology, University of Edinburgh*

Candace Currie BSc PhD Research Fellow; *formerly Research Fellow, Department of Zoology, University of Edinburgh*

Sonja Hunt BA MA PhD FRSH Senior Research Fellow; *formerly Associate Professor, Institute for Leadership Studies, Fairleigh Dickinson University, New Jersey, USA.*

David McQueen BA MA ScD Director; *formerly Associate Professor, Department of Behavioural Sciences, Johns Hopkins School of Hygiene and Public Health, Baltimore, Maryland, USA*

Claudia Martin MA PhD Research Fellow; *formerly Research Officer, Institute for Social Studies in Medical Care, Hampstead, London*

Erio Ziglio BA PhD Research Fellow; *formerly postgraduate student in the Department of Social Administration, University of Edinburgh*

Contributions to Chapter 8 were made by **Jane Jones, Community Worker on the Granton Health Project,** *who not only wrote part of the chapter but is largely responsible for the activities described therein.*

The views expressed in this book are those of the contributors and should not be taken to reflect the policies or perspectives of the major funding bodies of RUHBC.

Preface

This book grew out of discussions between members of the core staff of the Research Unit in Health and Behavioural Change and a collective concern, albeit from several different perspectives, about the emphases, methods and models which predominate in research and practices associated with health promotion and health education.

Although there do exist voices of dissent, health professionals, policy-makers and politicians have largely succeeded in promoting the view that individual behaviour is both the prime cause of ill health and a major factor in the maintenance and attainment of good health. This view has been reinforced by the media and has entered the domain of 'public facts' with very little critical debate about its scientific basis.

The authors believe that public health is about social systems and collective decision-making rather than being exclusively about the isolated activities of individual members of the public. It is assumed that concepts of what is desirable, in terms of public health activity, whether in individuals or in societies, are not absolute, but depend, rather, upon the perspective of the observer.

The dominance of certain groups, including members of the medical profession, administrators in the health field and the initiators and funders of research, in the definition of health needs and health problems according to their own criteria has created a serious imbalance in the type of research being carried out, the quality of the information available and the policies which have been adopted to address health issues.

The intention of this book is to examine the context and meaning of the behaviours, concepts and practices, both lay and professional, which may be pertinent to the public health and to relate these to the social structure within which they occur. The content is aimed at those people who are involved with community health and development, preventive medicine, health promotion and health education whether as researchers or as practitioners, medical sociologists, health psychologists, social administrators, health planners, policy-makers: all those who are concerned with issues impinging upon the public health. The book is written from a multidisciplinary perspective and is, therefore, more eclectic than other books on similar topics. Whilst not eschewing 'ideology', the material incorporates foundations for the application of methods and theory at a practical level. By its very nature the book is bound to put forward a particular viewpoint. However, pains have been taken to support this with a reasoned assessment of the available data.

We hope that this work will play a part in both supporting and stimulating critical inquiry into the present state of the public health, its antecedents and its amelioration.

Acknowledgements

We are very grateful to our secretarial staff, Beatrice Robertson and Emmanuelle Tulle-Winton, who, as always, remain calm, congenial and efficient in the midst of lunacy. Thanks are also due to Carla Zaccardelli for her assistance with the typing. Many thanks to Jane Hopton for her editorial comments and wizardry with the word processor, and to Margaret Christie for producing the index.

Introduction

Public Health, as a concept and as an activity, is wide-ranging. It represents an organised response to the protection and promotion of human health and encompasses a concern with the environment, disease control, the provision of health care, health education and health promotion. This book, written by staff members of the Research Unit in Health and Behavioural Change, is certainly not a textbook of public health. Rather it is a perspective on changing the public health, a perspective which is drawn from the social and behavioural sciences, rather than from medicine. It focuses primarily on factors relevant to health promotion in its broadest sense. It is not intended as a comprehensive review, but rather is an effort to redress what are regarded by the writers as serious imbalances in theory, research and practice.

The strategies of conventional health education are firmly rooted in a medical model which places the individual at the focus of intervention. Thus, changing individual behaviour is seen as the key to prevention of health problems and to improvements in the public health. Health promotion appears to hold greater promise because of the broadening of target areas to include professional practice, policy-making and socio – environmental issues. However, in practice many activities carried out under the rubric of health promotion are still focused on lifestyle, which may be easily interpreted as being synonymous with individual behaviour. Academic disciplines concerned with public health issues, such as community medicine, have also increasingly come to rely on models which recreate a clinical approach to disease in the guise of population measures. A focus on individual members of the public as agents of their own health status therefore permeates most current public health initiatives. The serious theoretical, methodological and practical limitations to this focus form the major part of this book. It is argued that to place primary emphasis on individual behaviour not only will be ineffective in reducing levels of disease, but also serves only to draw attention away from those social, economic and environmental conditions which create vulnerability to disease and illness in the first place.

The use of clinically oriented epidemiological studies to investigate the aetiology of disease has led to an undue tendency to seek explanations in terms of disease-specific models. Moreover, this view has come to dominate both professional and lay views of reality, even though its empirical base remains controversial and, in some cases, is very weak.

In general, levels of disease are comparatively low in Western industrialised nations, with increasing longevity and fairly high levels of physical well-being. The majority of diseases and the highest all-cause mortality rates are found disproportionately in the least affluent members of society and tend to cluster in areas of deprivation and disadvantage. Changing the habits of the people who live in such areas, even if it were to be successful, would do little to change overall levels of health, since the conditions which gave rise to the problems in the first place would remain.

The content of the book emphasizes the way in which certain themes have come to be dominant in the social construction of reality in relation to health and disease and develops the theme of why social structure is a more fitting target for change. Throughout, the term 'health' is regarded as a hypothetical construct for which there is no true referent in physical or emotional experience. In general, ideas of 'positive health' are eschewed; in part because of difficulties of definition and consensus, but also because such a notion lies outside the competence and strategies of would-be public health reformers, falling more within the provenance of the priest, the rabbi, the sports teacher or the psychotherapist.

The term *disease* is used in accordance with a medical model to denote deviations from 'normal' functioning in the clinical sense. Distress and illness are regarded as subjective states or processes which may or may not accompany medically diagnosed conditions, but which are indicative of the presence of suffering. The word *sickness* denotes social behaviours associated with illness and disease.

Behaviour is taken to be activity of some kind and may apply both to individual actions and to the actions of groups and organisations. It does not stand, as is often the case in the literature, as a synonym for 'attitude' which is taken to be a post hoc rationaliz-ation. Nor does the term behaviour necessarily imply a cognitive accompaniment.

Chapter 1 begins with a review of the history of the concept of health-related behaviour within developments in public health, social medicine and community medi-cine. The emergence of epidemiology as the favoured technique of these disciplines, the need of its practitioners to adhere to clinical-style explanations and the culmination of this in the risk factor concept, are described. It is argued that theory and research from the social sciences led to a widening of conceptualization in the field of health-related behaviour and that this has been largely responsible for putting the public back into public health and refocusing on social context. However, there still exist significant barriers to this viewpoint and health education and promotion remain dominated by a biomedical model. The second part of the chapter provides an overview of theories of behaviour stemming from diverse traditions, but with an emphasis on their use in theories of health-related behaviour. Many approaches to changing behaviour are predicated upon rational models of human action and have involved a knowledge-attitude-behaviour model. These are criticized for their lack of predictive and explana-tory power and for their failure to provide a societal perspective. The chapter concludes with suggestions for a more integrated approach to health-related behaviour which places individual behaviour in its social, economic and political context.

Chapter 2 focuses on some current issues in methodology which have particular relevance in data-gathering pertinent to changing the public health. Research in health-related behaviour has been dominated by ideologies and methods which originated in public health and the mainstream social sciences. To a great extent this research has followed the classic designs of the natural sciences, with a marked dependency on survey techniques, quasi-experimental designs, case control studies and other static designs. The limitations of these approaches are explored and the need for dynamic designs, as well as the integration of qualitative methods is emphasized. Positivistic approaches have been predominant possibly because of an underlying belief in the stability of human behaviour. However, such methods will not easily detect change and a longitudinal or panel design is usually deemed necessary for this. Some new data collection and analysis possibilities are described which may be applicable to the study of change, particularly through the continuous collection of data, utilizing mathematical, rather than statistical, techniques. The chapter concludes by arguing for more attention to be paid to the usefulness of computer technology and causal modelling.

The next chapter shifts the focus onto the social construction of health, illness, disease, and health-related behaviour. The cross-cultural diversity of beliefs about health and illness is illustrated by examples from cultural anthropology, and the growing body of work which examines lay perspectives of health and behaviour is outlined. From this it becomes evident that healthy and unhealthy behaviours have no absolute referents, but vary both between and within cultures. However, any formulation of health-related behaviour as directly reflecting cultural expectations and structural constraints must be inadequate and the chapter goes on to examine the everyday social processes and contexts within which behaviour takes place. This approach emphasizes the meanings that individuals construct as they attempt to make sense of and adapt to the experiences encountered in their daily lives. These meanings are developed and negotiated in interaction with others. Finally, the contextual and situational exigencies involved in the development of behaviours which relate to health and disease are analysed.

Chapter 4 describes the role played by both the press and television in conveying information about disease, illness and health, in relation to ideas of causation, treatment and prevention. It is maintained that the media represent a set of forces which present and reinforce dominant social constructs. In addition, they tend to support prevailing political trends and thus purvey messages which are unexamined in any critical sense. The content and form of the press are contrasted with those of television in the reporting of health issues. The role of the media in creating a climate of opinion is discussed and research studies reported which assess the degree to which the media can affect public opinion and comprise a factor in behavioural and social change.

The following chapter presents a new theory of health-related behavioural change, which is currently undergoing hypothesis testing. The chapter begins with a review of current models of behavioural change and some assessment of their performance in practice. It is argued that, in the main, these are without a firm theoretical base and neglectful of context. Many behaviours which may be associated with a health risk have a routine character, a habitual aspect which places them somewhat outside full consciousness. It is suggested that it is only when this routine behaviour is made salient that the possibility of cognitive appraisal arises. For such appraisal to be followed by change it must, however, take place within a relevant context, persist over time and include some notion of the opportunities for change which are available, as well as alterations in selective perception.

Evidence to support the theory is presented from work in neurophysiology and cognitive psychology, linguistics and animal behaviour. The role of behaviour in relation to adaptation is discussed and some postulates of the theory are suggested. Finally, the theory is used to show that it can be predicted that changes in behaviour will be least likely where certain prerequisites for change are not present, by reason of the social and economic circumstances in which people exist.

Chapter 6 reviews the data on social inequalities in death, disease, distress and sickness as they are traditionally measured. The explanations which have been given for these differentials are described and it is argued that if individual behaviour is a major factor in health inequalities then two propositions must follow: that such behaviours are similarly distributed in the population and that they do indeed constitute major risk factors. These propositions are examined in relation to smoking, alcohol abuse, exercise and diet. It is concluded that some behaviours may act as markers for the presence of distress or for particularly adverse socioenvironmental conditions rather than as major causative agents, and that others are likely to be be less significant than the structural factors which militate against the presence of good health in deprived and disadvantaged communities by creating a general susceptibility to disease.

Psychological distress, indicated by problems such as depression and anxiety, is prevalent in many populations, particularly in women from the working classes. Chapter 7 outlines the evidence which suggests that the principal antecedents of poor mental health are social. For example, people living in adverse housing conditions, the unemployed, those without supportive relationships, those with financial problems and women isolated with young children are all more likely to report poor mental health than are people in materially and socially secure situations. Structural explanations for psychological distress are considered in terms of their implications for a public health perspective involving social rather than medical intervention. More appropriate preventive services are felt to include improvements in basic living conditions, the provision of nursery facilities, self-help groups and locally based advisory and 'drop in' facilities.

Previous chapters have argued that attempts to change individual behaviour are largely ineffective, encourage victim-blaming and are particularly inappropriate under conditions of social deprivation. Theoretical and practical issues pertinent to health problems, their prevention and amelioration are brought together in Chapter 8 which describes a community development project in a deprived area of Edinburgh. The project is based upon community participation and the articulation of needs and problems by local residents. The processes of initiating such a project are described, with case studies of the various activities. An analysis of problems, conflicts and confusions is made, including an examination of the reasons for the opposition of some professional people to such projects. It is argued that such an approach can maximize the potential of the participants, create means whereby local people can have a voice in policy decisions and raise the general level of morale such that feelings of powerlessness are diminished and a sense of well-being is engendered.

Chapter 9 argues that the health impact of policy decisions is overlooked in the policy-making process. Moreover, the lack of coordination at the level of policy-making means that one agency may be trying to encourage one form of behaviour at the same time as another department may be acting to discourage the same behaviour. The term *health promotion* has recently come into vogue and is the focus of initiatives by the World Health Organization. Health promotion is distinguished from health education for its wider perspective and incorporation of socioenvironmental concerns. It is suggested that the ambiguity associated with the usage of the term health promotion may militate against it having any influence on policy. The lack of clear definitions of health also poses problems for the formulation, development and evaluation of health promotion strategies. It is against this background that the chapter sets out to provide a clearer understanding of the potential value of health promotion in tackling some of the problems raised in this book. It emphasis some uncertainties in intersectoral decision-making in the development of health promotion policies.

In the final chapter the themes of the book are brought together in a critique of current health education and health promotion concepts and strategies. The ways in which social problems are defined and explained are described as a function of the selection and distortion of information which enters the public domain. Attention is drawn to some serious gaps in our knowledge of factors which may affect the public health, e.g. the decisions of industrial organizations and corporate interests. It will be argued that current health problems require a reorientation on the part of professionals, policy makers' and researchers towards a genuine public health approach which targets structural factors at a population and community level as suitable cases for intervention. It is suggested that an alliance of professionals, research workers and lay people at local level can lead to the sharing of skills and knowledge, the raising of issues of local concern and the provision of hard data with which to back up demands for change at the level of public policy. Further research needs are described.

CHAPTER 1

Health Behaviour and the Public Health

Relevance of 'Health Behaviour' to Public Health

The Introduction to this book has briefly characterized the definitional problems associated with the words 'health' and 'behaviour'. An understanding of these two terms must play some part in the notion of changing the public health. Often the words are combined as 'health behaviour', further compounding the difficulties of definition. None the less, the term persists and has become commonly used in a variety of combinations: 'health-related behaviour', 'unhealthy behaviour', 'health-enhancing behaviour' 'health-damaging behaviour', 'health-maintaining behaviour' and so on. These terms and others like them are sprinkled heavily throughout World Health Organization (WHO) documents, health education reports' and in the daily press.

Problems with definition abound in the literature on health behaviour. For heuristic purposes, individual health behaviours may be divided into three 'types'. Roughly categorized, 'health-enhancing' behaviours correspond chiefly to behaviours concerned with health promotion, that is, those behaviours which are consciously undertaken in the hope of improving one's level of overall health. The use of the term health enhancement' has been widely adopted by WHO and many researchers concerned with the area of health promotion. A full explication of this terminology and its historical development is found in several chapters of a recent handbook on health enhancement (Matarazzo et al., 1984). 'Health-maintaining' behaviours are generally conceived of by health professionals as behaviours related to prevention. Many such behaviours are often independent of the formal medical care system, e.g. self-care and the routine use of vitamins; others, such as immunization and screening, do require limited interaction with organized medical care. Finally, 'health-damaging' behaviours include those which could be considered as negative health behaviours, such as the traditional 'risk factors' for disease, smoking, drinking, drug abuse. As is very clear in these definitions, health behaviour is seen largely as a property of individuals and such definitions lack any sense of applicability to collective behaviour. None the less, it is quite possible to reconceptualise many of these definitions as properties of social systems. Groups, organizations and even governments may be seen as engaging in health behaviours.

This chapter offers some views and speculations, if not necessarily answers, to the questions which arise from the diverse conceptualisations of health behaviour. Two broad approaches are taken: the first considers the historical development of the concept in Western industrialized societies; the second assesses the relationship of health behaviour to theories of behaviour in general.

It has been the bane of many pedestrian histories that the first appearance of words, e.g. 'health behaviour', has been considered sufficient to establish the origin of a concept or an idea, as if these symbols were, by themselves, the concept itself. Unfortunately, this type of misunderstanding is all too characteristic of writings in the history of medicine which have seldom dealt with underlying epistemological questions. However, the poverty of much historical tradition in the social sciences is also well appreciated; perhaps it is a sign of a young science, too early in its development to examine its past. It is because of these limitations that the first part of this chapter must remain somewhat speculative. There are few secondary sources on which to build a confident answer to the question, 'What is health behaviour?'

When searching for an explanation of the concept of health behaviour, there is rich resource material concerning human and animal behaviour which has been developed in zoology, ethology, psychology, sociology and anthropology over the last hundred years. Indeed, the behavioural sciences provide many of the underlying models of behaviour which may come to be adopted by those interested in 'health behaviour'. One of the strengths of research into 'health behaviour' has been its eclectic nature, the ability to pick and choose from the many behavioural models extant those which are most appropriate for health, even though the borrowed models have tended to favour some disciplines, notably social psychology, at the expense of others, notably zoology.

Part I: Historical Development of the Concept of Health Behaviour

The biomedical perspective

The biomedical perspective which provides one background and framework for current notions of health behaviour is represented by several histories, namely the histories of public health, social medicine, community medicine, behavioural medicine and epidemiology. In contrast to the vast literature on the history of medicine, histories concerned with public health, or which touch upon the public health, are very few. Undoubtedly this is the result of two key factors: (a) the relatively low status which public health has been accorded by the medical establishment; and (b) the fact that the bulk of medical history has been written by physicians interested in describing the development of modern medicine. The tradition of medical history writing in America, Germany and Britain has been dominated by medical-historical institutions which maintained a policy of allowing entrance only to qualified medical doctors. Thus, the major emphasis has been one of tracing the origins of the twentieth-century biomedical establishment, with particular emphasis on delineating the development of modern clinical medicine. Even distinguished medical historians, most notably George Rosen (1958), who turned their attentions to a history of public health maintained a powerful biomedical perspective.

Rosen's work remains the most comprehensive history of public health to this day.

His fundamental concern was in tracing, from ancient to modern times, a public health orientation to housing, sanitation and communicable disease. He presents a picture which encompasses the Graeco-Roman emphasis on water and sanitation, the medieval emphasis on epidemics, the Enlightenment's emphasis on disease prevalence, the industrialization period's emphasis on working conditions, and the modern era's emphasis on bacteriology and virology. Within these diverse time scales he documents a medical concern with the public's health, but seldom from the public's perspective and rarely from a non-medical perspective. In the Foreword to Rosen's history, Marti-Ibanez makes the point that the history of Public Health is therefore the story of man's endeavours to protect himself and his community against disease (Rosen, 1958, p. 14). The content of Rosen's work is largely the history of eminent physicians and their personal efforts to contain diseases stemming from environmental influences. Thus, his analysis does not focus particularly on the social contexts in which these physicians worked, nor on the social milieu of the time. It is not surprising, therefore, that a notion of health behaviour stemming from individuals or groups within the societies discussed is very much absent.

It could be argued that the public health movement, which had roots in larger social problems such as housing and sanitation, began with a 'social conscience' which continued into the twentieth century. Recent British interpretations of the development of public health within the biomedical perspective have located the initiation of the modern public health movement in the work of Chadwick and Simon (Chave, 1984). Chave traces the continuation of this movement in the Medical Officer of Health. He views the medical officer of health as the integrating figure who carried public health forward until the elimination of the post in 1974. But from the standpoint of the changing emphasis in public health from the societal to the individual, the history of the medical officer of health presents a very mixed picture. In general the focus of public health attention would gradually swing to personal health and hygiene during the mid-twentieth century. This would ultimately result in individual behaviours being identified as causally related to the principal chronic diseases of Western industrialized societies, namely coronary heart disease, cancer and a host of infirmities associated with the ageing process. These were the roots of a notion, which was to become very prominent in the 1970s of health hazards located in individual behaviour. Nonetheless during the period prior to the founding of the National Health Service, the Medical Officers of Health had gained considerable powers related to the public health, in terms of overseeing environmental services and problems, including housing, and, increasingly, the surveillance and control of infections and sexually transmitted diseases.

Lewis (1986) has discussed this controversial role of the medical officers of Health in great detail; what emerges is a discipline struggling to define its goals. She writes:

> The evidence suggests that MOsH neglected many aspects of their duties as community watchdogs during the 1930s, in respect both to more traditional areas such as immunization and to the new-found concerns over the effects of long-term unemployment on nutritional standards and levels of morbidity and mortality. In large part this neglect may be attributed to the narrow conception of public health as medical service and administration that characterized the thinking of MOsH during the 1930s. (p. 30)

Perhaps the demise of the concept of public health in the tradition of Chadwick began with the establishment of the National Health Service and was finalized with the elimination of the post of medical officer of Health in 1974. This view is strongly substantiated by Lewis (1986). She argued that the period from the end of World War I to post World War II witnessed both the failure of public health to develop a sound theoretical base and an increasing commitment to the provision of clinical services by the medical officers of health. These two characteristics formed a very weak base for a strong public health.

The public health movement which stemmed from the 'social conscience' perspective may have slipped away from the medical officers, but it has been argued that social medicine, and later community medicine, picked up the main themes and carried them forward. Chave (1984) makes this point:

> So we come to the night of Sunday 31 March 1974. On that night, the medical officer of health, the local health officer whom we had had in England since 1847, passed into the pages of the history book. And on the following morning there arose out of the ashes, like the Phoenix, the community physician. That day marked an end and a beginning. It marked the end of a system of public health that went back to the Royal Sanitary Commission and beyond that to the founding fathers, John Simon and Edwin Chadwick. It marked the beginning of a new system in which the community physician would occupy a key role within the structure of an integrated health service which offered comprehensive health care for all the people. (p. 16)

Essentially, this new integrated health service represented a further medicalization of public health. It signified that health, and even the wider context of health, was located within a health service primarily concerned with care and the delivery of services which were, in theory, designed to cure patients. One consequence of this decision, whether intended or not, was to place the focus of health on individual, or personal, health. From this orientation it was only logical that public health would begin to emphasize changing individual behaviours in relation to their potential impact on the health care system. With hindsight this new emphasis on the individual was unfortunate but foreseeable. Furthermore, it would be highly unfair to isolate and therefore give undue emphasis to the British situation. Similar trends were occurring elsewhere, particularly in the United States. Obviously. these trends cannot be separated easily from the broader issues of social policy which are discussed in detail in Chapter 9, nonetheless, a major effect was to lessen the concern with the role of social factors in health and illness and to place emphasis on individual psychological factors in health and illness.

The change in emphasis is fundamental, because of the implication of *what* it is that public health should try to change in order to improve the general health of the population. The focus moved away from the social environment, housing, work, income' and macro factors, towards coping, stress, social support, healthy lifestyle and activities located in the individual. The locus for change which might improve the public health had clearly shifted to the person and away from society. Thus, the very hallmark of the public health tradition from the nineteenth century was eroded. The strengths of a population-based, socially aware, public health with its concomitant methods and strategies were partly lost and largely replaced by methodologically weaker approaches which focused on individual behaviour. As Lewis argued (1986):

> But there was also a sense in which academics in the field believed that public health had 'lost its way', having been diverted into the provision of personal preventive services during the early twentieth century. When the Faculty referred to the specialty's origins, it usually mentioned the nineteenth-century pioneers rather than

the pre–1974 health departments. In 1981, for example, the journal *Community Medicine*, referred to the views of Sir John Simon, who 'looked forward to the day when "statecraft and medical knowledge took counsel together for the health of the people". and argued that the phrase could be applied to modern community medicine. A majority of academics were strongly convinced that the pre–1974 public health departments could not be defended and that public health had to be reformed and revitalized. The hope was to raise the status of public health by providing a more rigorous training for community physicians based on epidemiology and to create a genuine specialty of population medicine that was immediately recognizable as significantly different from general practice and hospital medicine. (p. 160)

It has been argued that the rising importance of, and emphasis on, community and social medicine were filling the breach left by the medicalisation of the public health. Social medicine already had firm roots in ventures such as the Peckham Health Centre in London, established in the mid–1920s. This centre would appear to have foreshadowed concepts of health behaviour which are associated with current ideas of 'of Health promotion-primarily, the idea that health was a positive social value (Pearse and Crocker, 1943). By the early 1940s the status of social medicine and preventive medicine had advanced to the extent that professorial chairs were established in Oxford and Edinburgh. Ryle, the first Professor of Social Medicine at Oxford, wrote in 1940: '. . . you must develop a social conscience, which has in the view of many of us, been too little evident in years preceding the war. . . I do ask you to be seriously interested in man's environment and the possibilities for its improvement' (p. 657). In many ways such a statement mirrors the health promotion ideology of the 1980s. What was remarkable about this earlier movement was the co-option of the word 'social' when in reality the curricula and training of social and community medicine in many medical schools remained largely devoid of the social sciences which stressed a broader view in harmony with a notion of social conscience (Rosen, 1979; Mackintosh, 1953). Instead, epidemiology dominated the curricula, and remains to this day the pivotal subject area of public health. This is not to deny that public health, whether found in schools of public health, departments of community medicine or departments of social medicine, is concerned with the health of populations, demography, public health administration, environmental sciences, the biological bases of public health, health services and public health practice, but most of these other areas are optional in the USA or alternatives in advanced doctoral-level public health programmes, or are covered in brief modules within 1 or 2 year masters' courses in Britain. Epidemiology remains the critical subject, without which the student cannot be regarded as 'properly cooked' in the public health perspective.

Epidemiology may be defined as the study of the distribution and dynamics of disease in human populations. Its purpose is to identify factors relative to man and his environment which influence the occurrence of disease and to provide a basis for programs in preventive medicine and public health. Epidemiologic methods are essential for evaluating the efficacy of new preventive and therapeutic modalities and of new organizational patterns of health care delivery. (Johns Hopkins School of Hygiene and Public Health, 1982, p. 103)

Public health is the application of the scientific disciplines to the resolution of . . . health problems. . . . It is imperative that public health base itself on scientific evidence. The range of sciences used extends from those specific to public health, such as epidemiology, to those shared with other fields . . . Epidemiology is the core science of public health and preventive medicine. (Detels and Breslow, 1984, p. 25)

The role that epidemiology has taken on in becoming the underlying discipline of public health, is a mixed blessing. Many would argue that epidemiology has brought a 'scientific' approach to contemporary public health. Within the social medicine component of public health, epidemiology is seen as the chief discipline as well. In his reappraisal of social medicine in terms of its contribution to social policy, Martin (1977) wrote:

> The pre-eminent concern of academic social medicine has unquestionably been the development of epidemiological methods and their application to the investigation of disease. Epidemiology involved direct access neither to the bedside nor to the laboratory; for the most part it took specific disease entities as its point of departure and could fairly claim to add a new dimension to clinical thinking. (p. 1336)

Perhaps one of the key reasons why epidemiology has occupied such a central role in recent public health and social medicine is that it encompasses a strong positivistic model of cause and effect. This has led to considerable concern with studying 'factors' underlying various chronic and acute disease processes. The social factor principle is predicated upon a notion of causality. Implied in the approach is the idea that some 'factor' causes a process to occur. Current methodological strategies in social epidemiology and behavioural science emphasize causal modelling. 'Causal modelling is a technique for selecting those variables that are potential determinants of the effects and then attempting to isolate the separate contributions to the effects made by each cause (predictor variable)' (Asher, 1976, p. 5). Indeed, in the last two decades this approach has led to a considerable body of research trying to explicate the role of sociocultural factors in chronic disease (McQueen and Siegrist, 1982). Many of these so-called 'factors' are seen as behavioural, e.g. smoking behaviour, eating behaviour, drinking behaviour. The difficulty, conceptually, has been to try to fit such 'factors' into a deterministic epidemiological model where it is almost impossible to make a sound case that these factors are determinants of disease rather than outcomes of other more basic sociocultural processes. In fact, one could argue that such behaviours are themselves mediating or buffering factors involved in complex social processes. The difficulties associated with specifying the place of behavioural/social factors in a positivistic epidemiological model underline the principal weakness of epidemiology as an approach to understanding health behaviour and, ultimately, changing the public health. A further difficulty with epidemiology as an underlying method for public health and research on health behaviour is its inability to handle multiple outcomes and multiple levels of behaviours, (McQueen and Celentano, 1982). Historically, many researchers have tended to ignore this problem and grouped many units of analysis together. Thus, data on individuals are simply aggregated into data on groups.

Futhermore the classic parameters of epidemiology (MacMahon and Pugh, 1970) namely time (disease occurrence), place (environment where disease occurs) and person (population affected), are very limited, especially in the assessment of a dynamic notion dealing with behaviour. That is behaviour, or better still behaviours, are not fixed at some point in time, but flow within a process which is extended over time, involving many 'places' (environments) and taking place within an individual's life span which is in continual development. In addition, disease or illness occurrence is not necessarily a measure of health behaviour. In the last analysis epidemiology is only a method, it has no underlying theoretical, conceptual basis other than a belief in the current scientific paradigm. Lacking a theory, it has no guidelines as to where to place human behaviour as a 'factor'; it may be a determinant, it may be an outcome, but only rhetoric serves as a guide.

The social science perspective

While it is undoubtedly true that a biomedical perspective has dominated public health in this century and thereby led to a medicalized interpretation of health behaviour, there has emerged, largely since World War II, a social science perspective into the public health debate. This perspective has developed in departments of community medicine (UK) and schools of public health (USA), and this growth is reflected quite often in the attention paid to the behavioural sciences in the curriculum. In North American schools of public health and to some extent in British departments of community health, this perspective has been seen in the establishment of departments or sections of behavioural sciences and health education.

The critical perspective of the social sciences fits uneasily into the biomedical tradition of public health. Negative judgements of the social sciences in public health are rarely publicly expressed or written down, but are often expressed in private and in off-the-record comments during meetings and on research committees. While not easily documentable, they are perceived as real judgements and are part of the folklore of fields like medical sociology. To begin with, the social sciences are regarded as 'soft science'. Indeed, 'hard' and 'soft' science are commonly used terms. This point is emphasized ever so painfully by the distinguished American philosopher-mathematician and, until recently, President of Dartmouth:

> It is certainly true that the physical sciences have developed to a stage far beyond that of the social sciences of today and even of the anticipated future . . . A typical law in the physical sciences is stated precisely, usually in mathematical terms, and is quite free of ambiguity . . . . The usual law in the social sciences, on the other hand, is ordinarily couched in Big Words [sic] and a great deal of ambiguity. (Kemeny, 1959, p. 244)

He later adds: 'But this stage, too, must pass. Eventually the social sciences will acquire a respectability matching that of the physical sciences' (p. 257).

It is important to emphasize this negative view of the 'social' sciences at the outset, because it is the fundamental prejudice under which every social scientist works when located in biomedical institutions. Social science, the soft option, is often held in reserve for when the 'hard' science, which in public health is epidemiology, cannot solve the 'scientific' puzzle. This helps explain, in part, why public health has incorporated such a limited piece of the rich social science perspective. Secondly, it is the very critical stance of the social science perspective which tends to marginalize the perspective. That is, it applies an evaluative, analytical approach to a field characterised by a medical view which asserts facts and answers to problems and often insists on 'solutions' which appear unambiguous. Thus, whereas a social scientist may wish to understand and analyse why such a phenomenon is occurring, the biomedical paradigm would conceptualize the problem in terms of 'diagnosis'. Indeed, in order to 'legitimize' medically their approach, many social scientists use the biomedical terminology as in the example of the 'educational diagnosis' of health education (Green *et al.*, 1980). Thirdly, the marginal position of public health itself, the belief that it is often a secondary career choice for medically trained individuals appears to place pressures on many public health practitioners to 'prove' biomedical legitimacy. The social science perspective does not often fit well into the desires of 'legitimated' recognition. Fourthly, the social science perspective encompasses a rich anti-positivistic theoretical tradition (Feyerabend, 1978; Foucault, 1973) which in many respects is anathema to the often rigidly positivistic orientation of biostatistics and epidemiology. Thus, much research in this tradition, particularly so-called 'qualitative' research, has grave problems of acceptability within public health.

There are many social science disciplines which are relevant to the understanding and articulation of health behaviour and its role in public health. In this brief chapter it would be impossible to consider the relevance of discipline areas as diverse as economics, history and anthropology. The focus must narrow to those disciplines which most directly attempt to describe, understand, predict and change human behaviour, namely sociology and psychology. In brief, sociology has argued for the influence of social structure on behaviour and psychology has centred on behaviour stemming from the individual's own brain. Obviously, these are gross descriptions; clearly social psychology has striven to provide an interactive person-environment explanation for behaviour, and sociology would hardly disregard the influence of individuals on structural patterns. What is remarkable is that the chief social science perspective which has come to dominate research on health behaviour has been social psychology with its focus on individual attitudes, motivations and practices. Why this is so will be considered below.

The general failure of public health and the study of health behaviour to pick up and nurture the more macro anthropological and sociological perspective has impoverished its development. Particularly so, because the social roots of public health in the nineteenth century began without a strong social-structural viewpoint. Since that time, the theoretical development of sociology and anthropology has accelerated, but it cannot be brought to bear on present-day public health issues because, increasingly, these issues are defined in terms of the characteristics of individuals rather than as characteristics of social structure. The argument is, then, that public health picked up the wrong end of the social science 'stick', i.e. the individual (micro) end rather than the sociocultural (macro) end. This assertion is easily supported by any perusal of public health journals or literature on health education. An example of this failure to engage the macro and instead, the continued support of the micro view is found in the so-called Health Belief Model, and that model serves to illustrate some of the points made above.

The seminal paper by Rosenstock on *Why people use health services* (1966) generated a considerable flow of health behaviour research during the late 1960s, throughout the 1970s and continuing into the 1980s. This outpouring centred on a notion termed the Health Belief Model, the underlying premises of which may briefly be described as follows: participation in matters relating to preventive health behaviour can be predicted on the basis of an individual's perceptions of: (a) his or her own susceptibility to a given disorder, (b) the seriousness or severity of the disorder, (c), the benefits of taking action, (d) the barriers to action and (e) cues to taking action.

The model was a heuristic device whose elaboration supported a plethora of research on the role of sociopsychological factors in both the seeking of care and compliance with medical regimens. It is not the purpose of this chapter to provide a literature review of this largesse for that has been adequately given elsewhere (Kirscht, 1974), or to elaborate upon the sociopsychological origins of the model, but rather to illustrate the inadequacies of the resulting research milieu. (There are other problems which are not dealt with here, viz: (a) the model considers primarily the 'negative' aspects of health behaviour, i.e. behaviour to avoid something deleterious; (b) the underlying motivation for action is not specified; (c) there are no sound operational definitions of the variables in the model; (d) the 'threshold for action' is not developed; (e) no consideration is made for attitudes towards the medical care system with which a person interacts; (f) confounding variables, e.g. education in particular, as well as sex, socioeconomic status, are not incorporated in the model.)

Despite the well-documented critiques of the model, it is widely applied in health behaviour research. Terms like 'perceived susceptibility' and 'perceived severity' fit well with an allopathic medical paradigm. The model has the appearance of social science couched in a 'scientific' language with meaning for medical professionals. Very thinly veiled in the model are the biomedical notions of etiology, symptoms and diagnosis. For example, the notion of 'perceived susceptibility' implies the idea of disease risk and 'perceived severity' the conceptualization of symptoms. Similarly the concept of 'cue to action' contains a kind of layman's self-diagnosis and early recognition of signs and symptoms.

The model was derived by social psychologists who rooted it in the work of Lewin. The term 'field theory', used primarily by Lewin and his co-workers, was an analogy taken from physics, where it conceptualized or modelled electromagnetic phenomena in terms of fields of electromagnetic forces. The parallel conceptualization of behaviour formulated by Lewin described a situation (field) in which a person participates. The model assumed that if one understood a person's situation, one would understand that person's behaviour, or movement within the field (Kirscht, 1974). Thus, Lewin's fundamental construct is that of behaviour occurring in a 'field', subject to change during a given unit of time. The field is consistent with the 'life space' of the individual, made up of the individual and his psychological environment. Rosenstock's interpretation of Lewin's formulation was that of 'an individual existing in a life space composed of regions some of which were positively valued (positive valence), others of which were negatively valued (negative valence) and still others of which were relatively neutral'. An individual's daily activities were to be conceived of as a 'process of being pulled by positive forces and repelled by negative forces' (Rosenstock, 1974, p. 330). In the Health Belief Model this interpretation is translated as: the avoidance of disease is positively valued and takes on a positive valence. It is postulated that a person who perceives himself or herself as susceptible to disease and views the disease as severe or having severe consequences will be pushed in the direction of taking health actions to reduce these threats.

Norman (1986) provides a careful and complete review of the strengths and weaknesses of the Health Belief Model. After a detailed review of the retrospective research and the smattering of prospective work on the model he concludes: 'In summary, despite its intuitive appeal, the evidence suggests that the Health Belief Model provides a weak basis for predicting or influencing health behaviour', (p. 62).

These criticisms are largely about the inadequacy of the model within a sociopsychological, personal behaviour perspective. It is apparent that such a model is also inad-equate if one takes a broader view of health behaviour, one that encompasses environmental concerns or that envisions behaviours at a group or organizational level. Neverthless, the field of health behaviour research has, in general, failed to provide alternative models to the Health Belief Model which have its apparent appeal.

Part II: The Relationship of Health Behaviour to Models and Theories of Behaviour in General

Part I of this chapter has illustrated one of the more common features of the study of health-related behaviour in public health, namely the desire to set up models to explain behaviour. The model which was used to illustrate this tendency, the Health Belief Model, is just one of many so-called models which have been put before researchers in public health and health behaviour. Although the word 'model' is often used in such research literature, it is generally used quite casually to explain a loosely held theoretical position. In fact, one could argue that 'model' is too strong a term and that some less rigid term such as 'idea-set' might more realistically describe these attempts to formalize ideas.

Classically in the natural sciences, models and theories have been the principal mechanisms put forward to provide explanation. However, it is important to acknowledge that the interplay between 'model' and theory has been of great importance for both the natural and the social sciences (Brodbeck, 1959). Historically, the use of models has often served as a mechanism to integrate several disciplines, as seen in the natural sciences where a series of useful models and analogies of atomic and molecular structure paved the way for common concerns in relatively unrelated sciences such as physics, chemistry and, more recently, biology (Achinstein, 1971). It could be argued then, that useful models in the social sciences may serve to bridge disciplines which have often divided the world artificially into individual versus aggregate behaviours and phenomena.

'Model' and 'theory' are two terms which are often used synonymously by social scientists. The usage of the term 'model' in logic, mathematics and 'hard' science may be more precise; there is a model for a theory which consists of an alternative interpretation of the same purely formal axiomatic system of which the theory is an interpretation. This is a fairly rigorous definition, probably too rigorous for social science; however, the empirical definitions of many social scientists may be too loose for practical purposes. If one takes the case of the Health Belief Model presented above, it would be difficult to discover how a formalized theory was being illustrated or articulated in the model. The logical adequacy of the model is decidedly lacking. None the less, few models or theories in the biomedical or social sciences are set up in such a way that their logical adequacy can be analysed. In the long history of research on human social behaviour, there is little theory or research which is presented in axiomatic form. Homans' work on social behaviour is a remarkable exception to this (Homans, 1961) and the logical adequacy of his work has been thoroughly documented by Maris (1970). Although this was pioneering theoretical work on human groups, it has not generated a large following in research concerned with health related behaviour.

Despite diverse definitions and lack of consensus in meaning, models are seen as 'good' things. Brodbeck, writing in 1959 on *Models, Meanings and Theories*, stated:

> The term 'model' appears with increasing frequency in recent social science litera-
> ture. We encounter models of learning, of rational choice, of communications of
> political behaviour, of group interaction, and so on, and so on. The term has
> moreover a decided halo effect. Models are Good Things. And if models are good,
> 'mathematical models', needless to say are even better. (p. 373)

Achinstein (1968) writes in the opening to a lengthy discourse on analogies and models:

> Philosophers as well as scientists tend to make sweeping and often confusing claims
> about analogies and models. Some accord analogies and models . . . a more central
> role in science than others; but all agree that these conceptions are frequently
> employed by scientists in the formulation and development of theories as well as
> for the interpretation of scientific terms. (p. 203)

In social science methodology, mathematical models underpin many current techniques (Huckfeldt *et al.*, 1982) and are particularly emphasized in log-linear models
(Knoke and Burke, 1980). in the area of socioepidemiological research, models of
association between stress and health have been actively explored (Marmot and Madge,
1987); this is particularly the case with research concerning psychosocial factors in
illness. Some recent examples are: (a) a casual model of the stress – illness relationships
(Kuo and Tsai, 1986); (b) a model of the effects of life strains on symptom patterns
(Newman, 1984); (c) a model of the effects of role-specific strains and stresses on
depressive symptoms and psychosomaticism in three daily social roles for women
(Kandel *et al.*, 1985); (d) models of hardship and depression (Ross and Huber, 1985);
(e) a multiwave, non-recursive causal model of depression and physical illness (Aneshensel *et al.*, 1984); and (f) models of sex differences in symptoms of depression
(Newman, 1984). In other areas related to the emerging public health, models appear
in such diverse concerns as: (a) a community coping with the threat of a hazardous
waste facility (Bachrach and Zautra, 1985); (b) gender and health (Verbrugge, 1985);
(c) planning preventive programmes in occupational health (Phillips, 1984); (d) infor-
mation-giving in medical care (Waitzkin, 1985); (e) and self-assessments of health by
the elderly (Stoller, 1984).

Because modelling is extensively used in current health behaviour research, two
specific examples are given here as illustrative; they well represent such research. In
the first example, Hayes and Ross (1986) report on the effect of exercise, being
overweight and physical health on psychological well-being. This study set out to
examine a variant of the ancient mind–body problem. In brief, they found that exercise
and good physical health improve psychological well-being, but that being overweight
has no effect; all of the observed effects were quite small. The study was based on 401
cases obtained by a telephone survey of Illinois residents; the main variables were self-
reported behaviour, weight and subjective sense of physical health. The 'standard'
sociodemographic variables were also obtained, e.g. age, marital status, education,
income, sex and religion. Hayes and Ross carried out the analysis in two parts. First
they evaluated social factors associated with exercise, overweight and physical health;
they conducted 'three regression analyses with each of the physical attributes as dependent variables' (p. 393). In the second part of the analysis they examined the interaction
among several variables in order to predict well-being; they argue: 'We interpret our

models in terms of the internal processes and social evaluation perspectives on the effect of physical attributes on psychological well-being' (p. 393). Thus, they used several alternative forms of causal models for their research. This illustrates the model form as a testing procedure which allows researchers to arrive at what they believe to be the best, mathematically satisfactory, model to explain the observed relationship. In performing their analysis in this way, they have followed a positivistic, scientifically derived approach in conducting social science research; thus their work well illustrates one use of models in health behaviour research, in particular that research which concentrates on individual behaviours.

In one area of public health, namely health education, models are widely used, but often without the same mathematical rigour as those mentioned above. The reasons for this are probably manifold, but their use in health education may well relate to some of the issues discussed above. To begin with, they may provide the field with some 'scientific' legitimacy and at the same time disguise the reality that health education has little theoretical basis. Secondly, the visual nature of models may be very sympathetic to the educational framework in which health education finds itself, i.e. they can serve as education tools for health education practitioners. Thirdly, evaluation research, which is often regarded as a pillar of health education research is generally conceived of in terms of quasi-experimental designs which, by their nature, structure health education interventions into an analogue of scientific models (cf. Cook and Gruder, 1978). Fourthly, the behavioural risk factor, epidemiological approach which is implicit in much health education effort is supported by the causal modelling approach discussed above. Finally, health education, particularly in attitudinal research on individual behaviours, notably smoking, has placed inordinate emphasis on explaining behaviour by psychosocial models (cf, Ajzen and Fishbein, 1973; Fishbein and Ajzen, 1980). More recently, health education has been joined by the idea of health promotion, a concept taken up in several chapters in this book. In the USA, health promotion has largely derived from health education as an area in public health and thus many of the same features of the parent, e.g. models and quasi-experimental designs (Green, 1984; Pelletier, 1987), emphasis on the individual (Jensen, 1987) are found in the offspring. The European experience has been different and had evidenced more societal emphasis, more eclectic methodology and a critical approach (Anderson, 1984; Tones, 1986; WHO, 1986a). Whether these differences in orientation will narrow or widen in the changing public health remains an open question.

As discussed above, models are often used in a very vague and less mathematical sense, sometimes more as a semantic device; the second example chosen illustrates this type of use in health education. Jensen's article entitled 'Understanding addictive implications for health promotion programming' *1987* is based on an examination of several models to explain addictive behaviour. She writes:

'Although such complex behaviours are clearly multiply determined, there appears to be good agreement that theories to explain addictive behaviour comprise three major categories: (a) disease model; (b) biological model; and (c) social learning model. (p. 50.)

After reviewing these 'models', she offers integrating models for the treatment of addictive behaviours and for programme planning by practising health promotion professionals. Jensen's article represents a very common use of models, but a very different one from that of Hayes and Ross. Rather than being a highly formalized, mathematical, causal form, this use is very casual. The word 'theory' could be interchanged with 'model' without any loss of meaning. In this application the value of a model lies in its use as a heuristic device for interpretation. This is undoubtedly because it seems easier to work with the seemingly concrete or visual (a model) than with an abstract theory.

Although not considered in great detail in this book, models of behaviour which have a basis in the biological sciences of physiology and animal behaviour are widely used in medical research, public health, medical sociology and behavioural medicine. These models are particularly prevalent in the prolific area of research related to stress and disease. In turn, stress research is a vast field which includes research into coping, life-events, social support, behaviour patterns, working life and 'hassles'. The size of this field is well represented in Hull's (1977) review of a decade of research on life circumstances and physical illness, and more recently in Kasl and Cooper (1987). In summarizing the content and method of 329 research articles Hull (1977) argued that: One of the clearest findings of the survey is that the social and behavioural sciences, particularly sociology and psychology, have not contributed in a major way to physical illness research in the last decade.' (p. 137). The underlying model in most of this body of research is sociobiologic (Henry and Stephens, 1977). That is, it assumes that social and psychological events which people experience, are experienced by the body as a machine, in terms of endocrinal and neuromechanisms. It is basically a mechanical model of disease (Sterling and Eyer, 1981) which is extended beyond mere internal physiological models to include the outside social environment of individuals.

In many ways this area of research well represents the ideal of multidisciplinary collaboration in research on behaviour and health. Many of the models proposed presuppose that the brain controls the physiology of the body; others emphasize environmental effects in setting up physiologies of chronic arousal accompanied by coping mechanisms. The critical public health question posed by such models is where intervention in this sociobiologic process can take place. This issue is well summarized by Sterling and Eyer (1981):

> The appropriate points to intervene in arousal-caused disease are not primarily at the physiological level, for the brain itself has the most delicate and rich systems for control at this level. It makes more sense, and will ultimately be far more effective, to intervene at the level of people's objective and subjective experience. It is necessary to understand what it is in their experience that generates and sustains chronic arousal. (p. 31)

Criteria for models in health behaviour research

Basically, there are two areas of concern as to the validity of a model: (a) the model must somehow be isomorphic with some underlying theory (of which the model is a more concrete realization), and (b) the model must be robust enough to withstand the same 'tests' as the underlying theory (thus one could argue that the same rules that apply to hypothesis testing with respect to some theory apply equally well to a model). Since a main aim of theory is to reveal order in seeming chaos there is often recourse, for heuristic reasons, to some sort of a priori model.

There is great risk in using models in health behaviour, risk emanating from several sources, but most importantly in the areas of isomorphism, and visualization and in the so-called problem of identification. The danger of non-isomorphism is self-evident; the danger of visualization is particularly relevant in the social sciences where the visual nature of many models – that is a diagram or figure, the convenient presentation of boxes and arrows – may lead the researcher to infer more from the model than from the implied underlying theory. Simply stated, the researcher gets carried away with the model itself. Finally, there are the dangers of overidentified models, where the model has more than one possible theoretical interpretation (very common in the social sciences), and unidentified models, where the model appears to yield results but there is no theory. Both these dangers are really the problem of isomorphism.

With respect to the use of models in health promotion and research into health behaviour, there is a need for some basic criteria to be met if they are to be salient. The first criterion is *contextualism*. This is not just the notion that the model works within a particular context, but the broader idea that the model should incorporate the context of the behaviour. That is, the behaviour is not simply determined by the context, but the two are inseparable. This criterion is implicit in many models of behaviour which have an ecological orientation. The second criterion of a behaviour model is that it must be *dynamic*: that is, it is capable of expressing states of behaviour at different points of time, characterized by motion and change. Although this might seem a logical approach to models of behaviour, it is very tempting to regard behaviour as stable and fixed with static parameters. Nevertheless, these apparent fixed or routine behaviours are still subjected to time and the minute changes of the ordinary daily life cycle. Thus, if one argues for routinization as part of a model, as in Chapter 5, that routinization is still a dynamic process. Part of this basic criterion of dynamism is the corollary that a model should be sensitive to changes in the life span. A final general criterion for a model of health behaviour is that it should be *interdisciplinary* in its content. It is too limiting to explain individual behaviour in terms of psychology only, when social or biological considerations may be just as relevant.

The development of new public health models of health behaviour requires that some basic questions be posed from a different perspective. For example, 'What contextual factors are related to population health behaviour?' or 'What health behaviours at the individual and societal levels are related to changes in the general health of the population?' The framing of such questions should be seen as an effort to abandon both the sociopsychological route with its focus on the individual and the biomedical view with its focus on disease etiology. In order to understand health behaviours it is necessary to view them at the societal level and focus the analysis on such corollaries as, 'Why do certain aggregates participate disproportionately in a given "health behaviour"? Stating the analysis at this level allows for the return to a middle range perspective which provides for the exploration of links between the social system and behaviours.

Conclusion

This introductory chapter has been necessarily wide-ranging, reflecting a belief that health behaviour is not rooted singularly in a medical perspective with emphasis on individual behaviour. At best, it has only hinted at the potentially rich background which health behaviour, and in turn public health, could find of relevance. The historical case presented argued that there were two chief derivations for health behaviour as a concept. The first, the biomedical perspective, was initially an area with a concern for the public health. Over time, this public concern placed more and more emphasis on individual behaviours as the focus for public health action. The social science perspective could have argued for a broadening of the increasingly individualistic medical approach, but the part of social science which was incorporated into public health focused on individual beliefs and practices.

CHAPTER 2

Methodological Issues

The methodology of research in public health is an enormous topic, therefore the focus of this chapter is limited to current issues in methodology which are prominent in health behaviour research, particularly in relation to changing the public health. An attempt has been made to consider those methodological issues which are either controversial or are currently seen as critical areas for further development.

Background

As pointed out in Chapter 1, research in health behaviour has been dominated by ideologies and methods which developed in public health and the social sciences. To a great extent this research has followed designs which have been well established in the natural sciences. Thus, there has been a marked dependency on the use of statistical techniques, particularly parametric techniques, resulting in a preponderance of surveys, quasi-experimental investigations, case control studies and other 'static' designs.

Perhaps because of an underlying belief in the stability of behaviours, positivistic, methods have dominated research in the field of health behaviour. However, such methods will not easily detect change. New directions in data collection and analysis techniques which may be applicable to the study of behavioural change, particularly through the continuous collection of data, need greater emphasis in public health research (McQueen, 1987b).

Methodological problems remain at the forefront of public health research because the ideology underpinning public health is often in flux. Ideas such as 'health promotion', 'community development', 'healthy public policy', 'lifestyle', either arise out of larger social movements or are rediscovered from time to time. The history of public health, even as reviewed briefly in Chapter 1 demonstrates that patterns of professional thinking may have relatively short time spans. Although ideas and rhetoric may move at a varied pace, they are highly susceptible to fashion. Fashion has always played a role in the history of science (Barbour, 1968) and public health is no exception to this. Although methodology used in public health is also subject to fashion, it could be argued that methodology: (a) changes more slowly, is often difficult to adopt, (c) is tied to hardware development and thus (d) develops at a very different rate from theory. To the first point it may be added that Karl Pearson's groundwork for present-day correlational statistics is now nearly a century old, but maintains a firm grip on the statistical paradigm adopted by public health practitioners (Porter, 1986). Even 'trendy' statistical methods, such as path analysis, owe their origins and methodology to genetic research and the work of Sewall Wright in the 1920s and 1930s (Wright, 1934). The mathematical and statistical techniques of social scientists such as Blalock (1969), Coleman (1964) and Tuma and Hannan (1984), which could provide innovative techniques for longitudinal analyses, are generally either not taught to public health scientists or remain locked in a narrow domain of methodological research within academic disciplines. Further, the mathematics underlying these newer techniques are not found in the training of most public health researchers because they stem largely from a mathematical theory base rather than from statistics. This is not to deny the mathematical and physical science basis of earlier statistical thought, but to enforce the notion that the earlier mathematical theory base has been generally disregarded by many practitioners in public health. With respect to the third point, the unprecedented development of computer hardware and software with its increasing 'friendliness' has allowed particular manipulative techniques to be applied with considerable ease to large data sets without any adherence to the mathematical assumptions underlying the techniques. Therefore, raw empiricism with large data sets is a path which health scientists can easily follow. Finally, this raw empiricism has brought about a lack of emphasis on the theoretical reasons for choosing subjects for study and fostered the proliferation of new variable constructs which arise solely from the manipulation of data, rather than from any substantive theoretical concern. This point is particularly emphasized in many techniques currently used, most notably in cluster analysis (Everitt, 1979).

The Issue of Research Design

The often discussed dichotomy of whether public health research should be qualitative or quantitative in approach well illustrates changing research perspectives. As a choice which can and perhaps must be made by the individual researcher, it is of note that some quantitative researchers view the qualitative approach of others with either disbelief or contempt, and vice versa, as if choosing sides in a political contest. The question is not which approach is correct; the research issue is how to move away from the simplistic notion that reality and, indeed, research can be so simply dichotomized.

The research issue is really the problem of 'linkage' (McQueen 1986b). If methods of research continue to consider reality dualistically, research must then be concerned with how the two 'pieces' relate to each other. That is, what are the rules of correspondence which link theory to observation, the qualitative to the quantitative, the individual to the societal? This remains largely an unexplored, unconsidered area for research, although recent encouraging signs are seen in the work of Tuma and Hannan (1984) and Fielding and Fielding (1986). Tuma and Hannan have taken the more mathematical approach, essentially making the point that both qualitative and quantitative research can be described mathematically and therefore equations derived from either approach can be set equal to each other. Fielding and Fielding have largely emphasized the multimethod approach wherein data collected by different methods are used to enhance a general picture of reality.

Discussions and arguments on the superiority of quantitative research are legion, particularly as championed by public health researchers seeking to justify the legitimacy of their work in a biomedically dominated setting. None the less, quantitative research, if it is to be meaningful, must be informed by equally good qualitative research. Having said that, one is immediately faced with the problem of how one actually does research which is combinatorial. There is an enormous literature on how to carry out quantitative research which relates to public health. Indeed, the entire methodological corpus of sociology, psychology and epidemiology may well be relevant. There is also a large body of methodological discussion in anthropology, history and sociology which considers techniques for qualitative research. As remarkable as the volume of this literature is the fact that very little beyond rhetoric can be found on combining these approaches. Furthermore, what does exist is usually written from the qualitative side of the dichotomy. Perhaps this is because qualitative researchers seek 'legitimation' through quantification; perhaps quantitative researchers are complacent in their assumed legitimacy ('Fat birds never sing'). Perhaps the fundamental problem is the continued acceptance of the view that there is a real, hard-fixed separation, instead of the shades of grey in the continuum between qualitative and quantitative methods. Given thought, it is hard to imagine how one can carry out public health research which is purely qualitative or quantitative and still consider it relevant or useful. If the ultimate goal of research is to reveal meaning, then it must slip easily back and forth from one approach to the other. In the long run the different approaches should 'converge' on some common understanding of reality; it is only in the short term that appearances of difference are revealed.

One of the principal problems in health-related research is that researchers may function as if there is a separation between theory and methods. Furthermore, the qualitative-quantitatve dimension often leads to the perspective that qualitative approaches are to theory as quantitative approaches are to methods. But why should this be the case? Such an argument would state that only qualitative methods could reveal theory. This is clearly too stringent a criterion to place on a theory. Indeed, some theories may primarily be illuminated through quantification; many sociological theories, by their very nature, express aggregate phenomena; e.g. social class is dependent on the quantifiable classification of an individual within a group. Nevertheless, one would not argue that social class is only a methodological trick with aggregate data. As a concept it has meaning and it has predictive power.

Type of research

One design issue concerns the type of research carried out in public health. The term 'research' is ambiguous by itself and is usually preceded by adjectives such as 'pure' or 'applied'. The difference between pure and applied research is also often unclear, some preferring the terms 'theoretical' versus 'practical'. Many other terms are used, e.g. descriptive research, evaluation research and, more recently, action research. In general, research concerned with public health is characterized as applied research, often more focused on description and answering questions as opposed to testing hypotheses. Thus, it is seen as empirical and objective. Emphasis is given to observables

– e.g. medical records, instrument readings – and 'indirect observables' – e.g. disease characteristics, signs, symptoms – over more abstract constructs – e.g. social support, coping-and highly abstract theoretically based terms – e.g. ego, social class. Where abstraction is high, the variables of interest are often made operational, ice. more concrete, by assigning values to abstractions, e.g. the Index of Social Position (Hollingshead, 1965) based on weightings of occupation and education.

Despite the considerable amount of emphasis placed on evaluation and research in public health, the meaning of the term evaluation remains rather unclear in this context. In general, evaluation research applies the same design strategies as applied research, although in many fields of public health, e.g. health education, it has come to be synonymous with the use of so-called quasi-experimental design (cf. Cook and Campbell, 1979). In recent years evaluation has been further subdivided into areas such as process evaluation and programme evaluation (Windsor, *et al.*, 1984). It is difficult to make a solid argument that evaluation research is anything other than rhetoric; that is, the touted strategies for research largely are an historical product of the 1970s tied to the rising concern and interest in demonstrating the effectiveness and/or efficiency of public health programmes. The research designs, particularly the experimental designs, were Baconian at heart, but glamorized to appear as a 'new' approach. Principally, the chief characteristic of evaluation research is that people other than the researchers define the questions to be asked and the goals of the study. In contrast, 'action research', seems not to have come from any 'classic' design for scientific research, although it does have analogies to problems and issues in twentieth-century quantum mechanics, especially with the principle that one cannot measure and predict in a system at the same time.

Action research is at present mostly an ideological stance towards research which argues that research should be active rather than passive. In traditional research, it is argued, the researcher is separated from and not responsible for the persons being studied. Action research eschews this separation. Thus, the course of a research project is not preordained in specificity, but only in general outline. This type of research will be discussed in more detail in the concluding chapter.

The Issue of Data Collection

The use of available databases

It could be argued that data collection in public health research is not always necessary, primarily because a large amount of data which may be useful already exists. This source of data is enormous in most industrialized countries and primarily consists of two types: (a) those which are collected routinely for government purposes, and (b) those which are the result of specific research endeavours, carried out by individuals, university research teams, private groups, etc. These data represent an immense resource for researchers in public health. Furthermore, data of the first type are generally descriptive information which has not been analysed further, and data of the second type have usually not been completely analysed because of the limited scope or funds of the researchers who initiated the study which collected the data. These data are often archived and relatively untapped: They are, however, generally computerized and part of the public domain, thus available to researchers interested in public health. Indeed, a review of studies reported in the *American Journal of Public Health* for one year (1985/6) revealed that 34% of them used computerized secondary data sources (Connell, *et al.*, 1987).

There are obviously many advantages to using secondary data in research. To begin with, data collection is a messy, time-consuming and expensive proposition. Secondly, because the data are computerized and ready to use, the researcher can concentrate entirely on analysis and can literally 'get into' the data very quickly. Thirdly, such data sets, particularly those which are derived from routine bureaucratic data collection, e.g. censuses, vital statistics, are politically 'neutral' and on face value are justified. Fourthly, because they usually come from legitimated data collection organizations, the data are often regarded as real, meaningful and accurate. For example, the Census is often viewed as a 'sacred cow', hardly capable of error; it is, after all, only collecting 'facts' about the population. Even secondary data which have been collected by academics take on a new legitimacy in that they are the fruit of an already vetted and approved study which has taken place.

Such secondary data are of marginal value for the changing public health because of both the quality of the data and the ideological underpinnings of the new public health. Firstly, the quality of such data is often their principal weakness. The data are primarily collected for administrative purposes, often by individuals who have little vested interest in their quality or consistency. Secondly, the purpose for which the data are collected is unrelated to subsequent use by other users. Mainly this means that the types of questions which would be of interest to a changing concept of public health are not asked during the data collection. Time and again, users of secondary data must stretch the meaning of questions to incorporate concepts which were never intended to be explored in the original data collection. This serious problem with the use of secondary data reveals the importance of having a theory behind the questions being asked. For example, until you have a theory of the role of some variable in a social process, e.g. a theory of coping, you cannot frame a meaningful question related to the social process. It is really quite unsatisfactory to go back to another set of data, collected without any notion of the social process currently under investigation, and expect to create the notion out of a set of other questions. Nevertheless this procedure is often practised in public health research using secondary data. As Johnson (1986) reported:

> A major difficulty in performing secondary data analysis is that the researcher must rely upon the questions posed in the original investigation. This study [The Impact of Workplace Social Support, Job Demands and Work Control upon Cardiovascular Disease in Sweden] would have been improved by the use of items and scales which specifically addressed job-related demand, control and support. This is not to suggest that the SCB's [Swedish Central Statistical Bureau] work environment questionnaire does not provide accurate and reliable data. But, the purpose of the ULP [survey of Living Conditions] was to generate a general portrait of the living and working conditions found throughout Sweden. It was not developed to specifically test the theoretical domains which have been the focus of this investigation. (p. 174)

The main strength of secondary data analysis is found when there is a strong isomorphism between current research questions and those of the past, ideally when identical or highly similar questions to those currently in use have been incorporated into the previous investigations.

Sampling

Sampling as a part of research has usually been guided by a need to satisfy rigid criteria established by statisticians (McQueen, 1987c). Indeed, this is often the only area of a research project where there are attempts to show rigid adherence to established statistical sacred cows. This may well be an artefact of the rudimentary training in statistical methods possessed by most social scientists working in public health; elementary statistical texts emphasize such concepts as randomness, normality and significance as paradigmatic items of research. Usually, this is at the expense of any sensitivity to the research problem being addressed. In fact, distribution-free statistical tests and procedures and their underlying rationales are rarely taught at the elementary levels despite the likelihood that the actual population research conducted later will largely be in violation of the statistical assumptions underpinning parametric sampling procedures. Thus, the key issue for the changing public health is how to legitimately break free from the rigid orthodoxy of sampling designs which are increasingly irrelevant to the special areas of study needed. To give a concrete example, if one wished to study a group of needle-sharing heroin users within a community in terms of their motivation to stop sharing, little substantial meaning could be added to the study if one had a random sample of such a group, presuming of course that one could even draw such a sample. This example merely emphasizes that it is the meaning, theory and purpose of the study which must guide the selection of the study population, and not rigid adherence to statistical dogma.

Continuous data and method

There are new data collection and analysis possibilities which may be applicable to the study of behavioural change-through the continuous collection of data. It is a challenge for the health research community to adapt to the new techniques for exploring continuous data which are becoming available just as it did to the traditional methods based on cross-sectional surveys which have dominated behavioural research. These new techniques will be able to detect certain types of behavioural and social change and will optimize longitudinal and/or panel designs.

Collecting data on a continuous basis presents many research issues which must be faced. From a technical point of view, the main issues revolve around sampling, data management, methods of data collection, and units of analysis. Sampling as a broad category has been discussed briefly above, but as an issue in public health research it presents some very basic questions in relation to continuous data collection. New methods of sampling need to be explored and should themselves be a subject of study. If, for example, the telephone is used, to continuously collect data and a random digit dialing technique is used, then sampling and information-gathering become coterminous. The solution of technical problems associated with such health behaviour research is fundamental to a 'dynamic' model of behavioural change. That is, most of the theoretical basis for sampling has been developed for static cross-sectional survey designs; in continuous data collection the sampling frame is never completed.

New problems have arisen in connection with continuous data collection. More emphasis has had to be placed on the 'mode' of collection. For example, telephone ownership is limited; mixed 'mode' methods, employing both face-to-face and telephone interviewing, have been developed. In general, concern has shifted to the problem of total survey error (Lessler, 1979) arising from sampling variability, non-sampling variability, response effects and non-participation effects. The latter is a special problem, as both American and European studies have noted an increase in non-response rates (Dalenius, 1977, 1979) for all types of interviewing. Many techniques such as call-backs, encouragement, substitution and promise of confidentiality have been used with varying success; in addition, statistical techniques such as weighting for missing data (Tupek and Richardson, 1978) and imputation techniques (Rubin, 1978; 1979) are being developed to account for data collection variability (Tanur, 1983).

The Issue of Measurement

The issue of measurement has always occupied a central place among the thorny problems of social science research, particularly the problem of validity. In a field that creates variables which often lack specificity and easily objectifiable measures this is bound to be the case. The ideas of most profound interest in public health, e.g. inequity, quality of life, perceptions of health, social stress, coping, enablement, deprivation, to name but a few typical concerns, are all concepts or social constructs. Even if one believes firmly that deprivation, for example, is a 'fact', its measurement, that is the assignment of a numerical value to its relative level, is exceedingly difficult.

To illustrate the measurement issue, consider the concept of 'health-enhancing behaviour'. Certainly, this is a concept which is widely used in current literature on health promotion. A quantitative researcher, faced with such a concept, would be concerned with how to measure it, and seek examples of what activities performed by people are considered, by health professionals, to enhance an individual's health. A list of behaviours would be assembled. This list would probably include such items as jogging, smoking, stress reduction, eating less fat, and so on. It matters less what is on the list than whether the item is quantifiable, e.g. how much fibre does X eat per day. In due course, following much discussion about the exact wording of the questions, several hundreds or thousands of people will then be asked to respond to the question, 'How many slices of whole wheat bread do you eat per day?' Thus operationalized and combined with other question, the researcher would have made an attempt to measure part of the construct. A qualitative researcher, faced with the concept of health-enhancing behaviour, would probably ask how the meaning of the concept could be revealed by talking with and exploring the idea with a rather small number of individuals, perhaps starting with some lines of inquiry about health in the most general sense. Only through a long-term process would the concept of health-enhancing behaviour be revealed.

Accepting that there really is something called 'health-enhancing behaviour', it is clear that these two research approaches will produce two very different pictures of the concept. It is also likely that they will produce two inadequate pictures of the concept. A meaningful, more adequate picture would be produced by linking the two approaches, that is by a team of researchers, using both methods in the same population, going back and forth between the two research strategies. This 'pendular' approach is, indeed, quite feasible. Starting first with in-depth qualitative views of individuals, a list which has meaning for the individuals and comes from the individuals is gradually constructed. Then the quantitative task is to design question items which recover these meanings in the same people. A more structured interview might then follow, but it should not mean the abandonment of the qualitative approach. Concepts and people, and their ideas of concepts, change over time and one must avoid the danger of quantifying concepts at an early stage of research and fixing in concrete that which is dynamic. The essence of such research is that it is concerned with process; the researcher can never feel that any instrument or approach has fully revealed the underlying idea being studied.

The problem of construct validity does not end with the measurement issue. Even if a proper indicator for a concept has been devised and there is general agreement that the indicator or index accurately measures what it is supposed to measure, there remains the problem of the data collection method and its effect on validity. Each method used to collect data, whether face-to-face interviewing, postal questionnaire or telephone interview may affect validity (Belson, 1986). The question of how validity may be compromised by method can only be answered by further attention to methodology; Belson commented:

> A number of comparative studies of the results from telephone and face-to-face surveys have been made. These indicate a broad similarity of results for the two methods, though there are some exceptions. But even when there is agreement, there is still a possibility that both methods are wrong in the studies concerned . . . . What is necessary for the safe use of the telephone survey method is that validity testing of it be carried out on a wide range just as is necessary for assessing the validity of the face-to-face survey interview method. Such validity testing would have to take into account different subject matters, different question forms, different contact rates and different refusal rates. (pp. 537–8)

Currently, a major issue in measurement in public health concerns the development of indicators. This is a task of high priority for the World Health Organization, particularly in conjunction with their Health for All by the Year 2000 programme (WHO, 1986). All the targets set by this organization are highly relevant to the changing public health but, in order to assess and evaluate the attainment of these targets, there is a need for outcome indicators. Many of these targets set goals for which indicators are highly objective, e.g. the assessment of infant mortality, or infant birthweight. Still other targets, particularly those dealing with health policy and healthy lifestyles, lack indicators which are agreed upon in the research community. The fundamental problem is one of construct validity, i.e. what is the indicator, or marker, for the concept. The difficulty goes to the heart of the philosophy of science in that there are no agreed-upon or clear-cut rules to spell out when an indicator has corresponded totally with a concept. The solutions to construct validity may not lie in methodological procedures alone, but in a complicated relationship between theory and methods. As was discussed in Chapter 1, many of the most relevant concepts in the emerging public health lack a strong theoretical base, thus creating a vicious circle which is not amenable to rapid solutions. It is unbridled optimism to believe that valid indicators of key social constructs will be forthcoming in the immediate future.

The Issue of Data Management

New methods of data collection have implications for the management of data. For example, in traditional survey research the period of data collection precedes the conversion of the data for analysis. Typically, questionnaires are stockpiled, then coded, and when coding is completed a finished data file is processed.

However, in order to study changes in behaviour and to account for periodic differences, one strategy is to collect data in short 'bursts' and, in the ideal case, on a regular basis throughout the year. The brief periods in between bursts can be utilized to review the data received to date and allow for strategical adjustments in questions asked. This 'burst' method of data collection requires a data management approach. Such an approach is conceptually more like taking an 'inventory', in this case an inventory of behaviours. Fortunately, the current state of computer technology makes such an approach feasible, especially with the possibility of daily on-line entry of data and the use of computer-assisted interviewing techniques.

Once individuals became part of such a study they would become a database for information on both long-term and short-term behavioural patterns. Thus, once interviewed, they could be re interviewed, by telephone, post or face-to-face methods, at regular intervals. Further, quarterly subsamples on special topics, with brief interviews, would be possible in order to assess changes resulting from some particular contextual phenomena, e.g. a government report on smoking or a national health education campaign.

This approach really implies that a study is always in process; it is never completed. It also implies that what constitutes a completed 'burst' or subsection of this long-term process is very much up to the researcher, particularly because the method for managing such data is not well worked out in the behavioural sciences related to health. There are other sciences which study units of data collected continuously, notably economics, physics and biology – models and methods from these fields need to be considered. In addition, much more attention needs to be given to the time dimension of data collection, not just in an emphasis on longitudinal studies, but with an emphasis on the management and analysis of this information. This is particularly important in the changing public health where the theoretical emphasis is on social processes. If lifestyle and context are to be taken seriously as theoretical ideas in health behaviour research then they must be seen as processes. As Tanur (1983) stated:

> People do not change jobs, break up marriages, and so forth, at specific (discrete) times (such as at the time they are asked about their status on these variables). Thus, any decision about the proper length of the time period to consider is necessarily arbitrary. Weekly is probably frequent enough to observe whether job changes occur-but is monthly frequent enough? And analyses that make these arbitrary decisions differently for use in discrete time models can produce substantively different results. (p. 34)

When time is introduced into the data collection/data management issue this has powerful implications for analysis, which will be discussed below. If it is change over time which is the subject of study then the fundamental question is the unit of collection. To date, most longitudinal data have emphasized the change in individual behaviour over time, concentrating both on real time and time in an individual lifespan. This, of course, tends to emphasize the individual at the expense of the collectivity. None the less, behaviours as phenomena themselves also change in character and structure over time and groups exhibit different behaviours over time. Despite the richness of longitudinal data collection, public health research has not addressed the collection and analysis of data on non-individual units.

The Issue of Data Analysis

There are many issues in data analysis related to changing the public health. Although data analysis, with the advent of new computer hardware and software, has become increasingly sophisticated, it has also resulted in a separation of analysis from the rest of the research endeavour; it has in fact, become a field within itself, increasingly remote from the behavioural scientist. This trend is rather unfortunate in that substantive issues may be overlooked in the rush to begin data analysis. Ever more sophisticated analyses may well obscure rather potent findings which need to be brought to the attention of workers in public health as well as to policy-makers. This section concentrates, for the sake of parsimony, on only two of the central issues in analysis which require attention if data analysis is to serve a meaningful role in the new public health.

Multiple units of analysis

One of the most pressing problems is that data in research on behaviours are often presented or collected at two or more levels of observation. Historically, many social science researchers have tended to ignore this problem and lumped all the units of analysis together. Thus, data on individuals are simply aggregated with data on groups. Often the 'levels' of the units are not conceptualized as different and such conceptual entities as 'individuals', 'households', 'neighbourhoods' are simply linked together as if they were, from a measurement standpoint, the same kind of unit.

Data are usually collected only on individual behaviours and self-reports or perceptions of social processes. Perhaps this is because the distinctions are not as conceptually clear-cut as units of analysis in the natural sciences (e.g. in biology-the molecular, cellular, tissue, organ levels). In addition, the statistical underpinnings of multilevel analysis (cf. Lindley and Smith, 1972) are beyond the scope of most social scientists. Recently, Mason et al. (1983) have made efforts to bring these analytical considerations to the attention of sociologists. The underlying strategy is 'the notion of a regression in which the dependent variable consists of regression coefficients from other regressions'. (p. 73). The use of such techniques in the study of behaviour related to health is worth consideration, owing to the fact that data are often a mixture of different levels. But such strategies, if they are to be employed, require a multi disciplinary and perhaps a multicentre approach (i.e. involving research centres with different kinds of expertise, and experience with different levels of variables). The future developments of such techniques may well be crucial to the very 'essence' of a changing public health.

Causal modelling in the new public health

Current research strategies in social epidemiology and behavioural science emphasize causal modelling [cf. Chapter 1]. The social factor principle is premised on a notion of causality. Implied in the approach is the idea that the 'factor' causes a process to occur. The statistical techniques for the required multivariate designs have been extensively developed in the past 15–20 years, pioneering work in this field having been conducted by Blalock (1964, 1968), Goodman (1973) and Land (1969). The coterminous development of computer hardware and software has facilitated the use of these techniques by social scientists, now seen in the common use of multiple regression, path analysis, log-linear analysis and Lisrel by social scientists (Joreskog and Sorbom, 1982; Alwin and Hauser, 1975; Kessler and Greenberg, 1981; Henry, 1982). Only recently, however, has attention been paid to such applications with discrete data (Feinberg, 1980; Goodman, 1984; Winship and Mare, 1983). The state of the art indicates the feasibility of such causal modelling for data on behaviour related to health; the question remains as to whether this wealth of methodological techniques can be integrated into health behaviour research linked to public health.

Analysis which is dynamic

This is the second main issue in analysis. As discussed above, there is increasing attention to data collection which is not discrete or static, but is dynamic. The result is the need for development of analytic strategies which can adequately analyse these dynamic data. Despite this need, the major emphasis in public health methodology still relies on the analysis of static relationships, particularly with the use of cross-sectional data. Even when panel or time series type data are studied, the data are still treated cross-sectionally, i.e by looking simply at the changes from one static state to another. Fortunately, within current data analysis literature, particularly that being developed in the USA, increasing attenton is being given to dynamic analysis. Although these techniques have been eloquently championed by Coleman, beginning over two decades ago (Coleman, 1964, 1968, 1973), they have not been widely used until recent years. The reasons for this are obscure, but may lie with the vogue of causal analysis research which accompanied more sophisticated technology. More recently, Tuma and Hannan (1984) have written a major treatise on the subject and this seems to have sparked considerable interest in the social science literature on such methods. This potent analytical approach, which seems to be well adapted to the qualitative and quantitative approaches needed by the changing role of public health, now offers new data analysis possibilities. In their Introduction they argue:

> Ample motivation for dynamic analysis exists; therefore the paucity of empirical studies of change in the sociological literature cannot be explained by its lack of worth. We think that the primary problem is methodological The literature on methods for analyzing data on change over time is both fragmentary and disorganized, and it tends to emphasize potential pitfalls of temporal analysis (such as autocorrelation bias) rather than to emphasize its advantages. Clear guidelines concerning alternative designes, models, and estimators are lacking. (p. 16)

Their work, along with that of others, provides a useful starting point for new methodological developments applicable to public health.

Discussion

As has been discussed, methodology is in itself a complex area of research which has consequences for the type of public health research which is acceptable among researchers. But the concern for methodological sophistication and use of acceptable paradigms has often led to reported research which has only a limited impact on changing the public health. This introduces the issue of appropriate methodology seen in terms of the potential users of the research: that is, what constitutes the appropriate presentation of 'evidence' of some finding related to the public's health. This issue cannot easily be separated from methodology as discussed here. There are two stumbling blocks: (a) presentation of research and methodology designed for other researchers and 'scientific' evaluators, and (b) presentation for international organizatons and policy-makers. The first group can be characterized generally as conservative methodologically, expecting 'classical' approaches with regard to data collection, sampling and analysis. The second group generally seeks readily accessible findings and emphasizes 'simple' methods which can be understood by the non-professional. These two positions would appear to be completely at odds with each other and at the same time present a major obstacle to the use of more appropriate methods in public health. Furthermore, the public health researcher has generally avoided the implications of this issue. Hence, many studies which could show promise yield grey documents which adhere to classical methods and are unread by those who could influence change. Finally, and most important, the real end-user of research is the public; this issue of the public use of research will be discussed further in the final chapter.

> The epistemological obstacles which social science has to overcome are initially social obstacles. One of these is the common conception of the hierarchy of the tasks which make up the sociologist's job, which leads so many researchers to disdain humble, easy yet fertile activities in favour of exercises that are both difficult and sterile. Another is an anomic reward system which forces a choice between a safe thesis and a flash in the pan, pedantry and prophecy, discouraging the combination of broad ambition and long patience that is needed to produce a work of science. Unlike the sometimes illuminating *intuitions* of the essay form, the sometimes coherent theses of theoreticism and the sometimes valid *observations* of empiricism, provisional systems of scientific propositions which strive to combine internal coherence and adequacy to the facts can only be produced by a slow, difficult labour which remains unmarked by all hasty readings. (Bourdieu, 1984 p. 512)

CHAPTER 3

The Social Construction of Health and Illness

Introduction

Historical and cross-cultural studies have demonstrated that concepts of health and illness, and their related behaviours, are complex products of the social groups in which they develop. Any discussion of changing the public health must, therefore, take account of the factors involved in the social construction of health and illness. This chapter will focus on the importance of cultural, phenomenological and interactional factors in the development of health and illness concepts and behaviours. The effects of social-structural factors on the public health, notably the distribution of political and material resources within society, are examined in detail throughout this volume. This macro perspective must be seen as essential background to the more micro concerns addressed in the present chapter. Factors such as occupation, social class, age, sex and ethnicity clearly have demonstrable effects on health-related behaviours at the population level. What is less clear, however, is how such factors are mediated through cultural norms, how they acquire meaning at the level of individuals and primary goups, and what are their practical implications for everyday health and illness behaviours.

Analysis of the social construction of health and illness may take place at different levels of abstraction. Firstly and most broadly, the individual's interpretation of his or her bodily state may be related to a search for purpose and meaning in life generally. Such a development of cosmology, or world-view, characterizes all societies, and goes beyond any form of medical explanation. For example, when illness strikes the individual, the questions 'Why me?' and 'Why now?' may demand explanations which transcend medical diagnosis and require examination of the social order or the order of the world generally (Herzlich and Pierret, 1986).

Secondly, however, the pluralistic nature of all complex and many simpler societies means that a single world-view is seldom accepted totally by all members. Thus, the social construction of health and illness must be seen as taking place in the context of competing cosmologies and power groups, as Unschuld (1986) has commented:

'Wherever, within a particular society, groups of different ideological persuasion co-
exist, we shall also encounter mutually exclusive systems of medical conceptualization. The question of which of these is predominant is resolved by the predomi-
nance of the world view (p. 54).

Moreover, Unschuld argued that fundamental social changes, and the concomitant
alterations in the world-view dominant in that society, will be accompanied by changes
in concepts of health and illness. For example, the foundations of the dominance of
Western clinical biomedicine were laid at the beginning of the nineteenth century,
coterminus with the rapid expansion of industrial capitalism and its associated social
change (Foucault, 1973).

Thirdly, and consequent upon these historical changes, particular groups within
society may attain the power to determine which form of medical conceptualizaton will
predominate. Thus, in developed countries, the biomedical model of health and illness
now predominates over indigenous medical systems and lay concepts. Whilst taking
different views of the derivation of biomedical dominance and how it may be challenged,
critics such as Illich (1975) and Navarro (1976) have claimed that the power invested
in scientific medicine now extends into many areas of social life other than those of
health and illness. Illich described a process of 'medicalization' whereby many life
experiences are increasingly subjected to medical definition and jurisdiction. Consequently, individuals increasingly define their problems in medical terms and look to
physicians to solve them. On a cultural level, a further effect has been that traditional
ways of coping, for example with illness and death, are being undermined. Navarro
viewed the power of medical groups as stemming from societal forces. Whilst scientific
medicine appears to be influencing significant decisions about individuals' lives, Navarro
argued that medicine itself is dominated by the capitalist system. Thus, notably in the
USA, profitability has become the main determinant of health care decisions.

Historical and structural processes involved in the social construction of health and
illness are recurrent themes elsewhere in this volume. The present chapter will,
however, concentrate on those analytical perspectives which demonstrate how health
and illness are affected by cultural factors; and how they may also be analysed as the
products of meanings negotiated in everyday interaction. The first section relies heavily
on the anthropological tradition to demonstrate the importance of cultural factors.
'Culture' has been defined in various ways. Donovan (1986) concluded that it:

'involves the beliefs and customs a society develops in attempting to manage its
shared problems; and (culture) orders 'proper' behaviour, priorities, social norms and
values. It is embodied in language, the primary form of communication; (and it) subtly and systematically affects perception and invests it with emotional significance. (p. 31)

The next section concentrates on research in Western societies and outlines how, first,
positivist and, more recently, interpretive approaches have addressed conceptual factors
involved in the social construction of health and illness. Stacey's (1986) reminder that
concepts are not neutral but embedded in social life and, therefore, associated with
actions taken, and given sets of social relationships, is pertinent. This applies not only
to lay concepts but also to those of 'allegedly neutral science' (p. 11); and Stacey
emphasized that, like their subjects, social scientists are creatures of their time and
place. Thus, the interpretive approach developed in part out of criticisms of the positivist
tradition and its arguable claims that quantitative methods were value-free and scientific
in the same way as it is supposed are those of the natural sciences. The interpretive

approach favours qualitative methods. The different groups subsumed under its umbrella all stressed that the main foci of study should be the subjective meanings, taken-for-granted assumptions, and social processes involved in the social construction of reality.

Drawing on these wider developments in social science, interest has grown in how individuals perceive, experience and negotiate meanings attached to health and illness. A final section describes and discusses the main themes in the body of work which examines the pluralism of lay concepts existing within Western societies characterized by a dominant biomedical system. Drawing on an analysis of the problems involved in these studies, some neglected areas of study will be outlined which, it is argued, should be incorporated into future research.

Cultural Influences on Health and Illness

Theory and method are interlinked in social scientific research. Therefore, in order to understand the re-emphasis in recent years on the importance of the sociocultural context of health behaviours it is useful, briefly, to examine established anthropological and sociological approaches. From this it is evident that in evaluating what is presently known about health and illness it is necessary to appreciate how the data were gathered and the assumptions and rationales behind the work.

Anthropologists have a long tradition of documenting the medical beliefs and practices of non-Western peoples. The early ethnographic works were designed to relate such practices to the particular culture under study (Evans-Pritchard, 1937; Rivers, 1924). The researchers were concerned to understand medical beliefs, practices and aetiologies from the point of view of the peoples concerned (an 'emic' approach). In the early ethnographic studies, such behaviours had their own intrinsic interest as items of culture, and the functions of health and illness, for example, were documented as expressions of broader cultural norms and values. Usually, the descriptive nature of these studies, relying principally on participant observation and qualitative methods, meant that the implications of these practices for the actual health of the peoples concerned were seldom addressed, (Foster, 1975).

Subsequently the work of medical anthropologists assumed a variety of forms. On the one hand studies continued to adopt an 'emic' perspective, characteristic of traditional anthropology generally. Such studies employed largely descriptive and qualitative methods. They concentrated on describing and, increasingly, analysing indigenous explanations of health and illness which had developed independently of the Western biomedical paradigm. On the other hand branches of medical anthropology such as epidemiology and medical ecology examined the distribution and aetiology of disease within the framework of western biomedical definitions (an 'etic' perspective). These studies employed mainly the statistical survey of populations. This methodology involves exploring associations between predefined variables or sets of variables on a population basis. This survey approach generally has been recently criticized by Coleman (1986). He pointed out that the end result is extraordinarily elaborated methods for analysing the behaviour of a set of independent entities (most often individuals), with little development of methods for characterizing systemic action resulting from the interdependent actions of members of the system.

Gradually, the practical clinical utility of medical anthropological knowledge became appreciated and this influenced the types of studies which were carried out, for example anthropological information was useful in understanding cultural change; or was seen as necessary for the effective implementation of Western medical programmes in developing areas (Foster, 1975). Wellin (1958) outlined the implications of local culture for public health: it affected the ecology of health and disease; it created its own subjective picture of health and disease; and it influenced the career of health programmes themselves. Thus anthropologists have documented illness and disease classifications and aetiologies, therapies, prophylactic measures and the role of folk special-ists in many indigenous cultures. The practical relevance of examining the implica-tions of local cultures for public health programmes persists, for, as Lieban (1974) stated:

> Yet for the most part both practitioners and the population at large dichotomize the medical situation in developing societies, competition between local healers and physicians is often intense, invidious distinctions abound, and differences that people perceive in the two kinds of medical systems can have a significant effect on the medical choices they make. Knowledge of the reasons for these choices not only has practical value for efforts to improve local, regional and world health, but also can contribute to a general understanding of human behaviour in relation to culture changes. (p. 1056)

More recently, anthropological skills have proved of clinical relevance within Western societies. Researchers have analysed and developed models of the contrasting lay and professional medical care systems which operate concurrently not only cross-culturally but also within developed societies themselves (Kleinman, 1978; Young, 1976).

In the past decade medical sociologists have been using qualitative and observational methods to a much greater extent. Traditionally, however, the main trend has been towards survey research and quantitative methods. In part the continuing acceptability of these methods can be related to the assumption that the western medical system was a non-problematical conceptual unity. The tendency of most medical sociologists to work within the biomedical model and to identify with the medical establishment, accepting their definitions of necessary research problems (Freidson 1970b), reinforced the assumption that there were shared conceptual frameworks between subjects and observers (Comaroff, 1978; Foster, 1975). More recent work has begun to redress this balance to look at health and illness as social processes (Fabrega, 1974, Fabrega and Manning, 1979; Dingwall, 1976); and to acknowledge that the study of emic definitions is of equal importance in Western and non-Western cultures. For instance, taking the example of ill health, Fabrega (1976) drew up a set of propositions in an attempt to develop a theory of human disease. These included the criteria by which social groups themselves defined a particular disease and the understandings lay people had about the disease as well as its behavioural and social effects, and the way the disease was expressed socially. In addition, structural factors had to be considered, such as the institutions which developed in order to deal with the disease, changes over time in medical orientation, and the success of dominant groups in controlling the disease according to their own definition. Once the pluralism of the Western health system had been accepted, many sociologists and anthropologists began to focus on the ways in which health and illness behaviour reflects power divisions, at macro and micro levels in society (Young, 1982; Frankenberg, 1980; Taussig, 1980; Navarro, 1976).

Finally, anthropologists have also demonstrated the cultural complexity underlying many everyday behaviours which have implications for health, illness and the public health. A good example of the ways in which cultural factors affect health-related concepts and behaviours is in the area of eating and drinking. This is especially pertinent in view of the current official reports on 'good diet' and the consequent exhortations to individuals to make changes in what they eat and drink to accord with nutritionally sound directives (NACNE, 1983). Not only is the relationship between diet and health controversial, as discussed in Chapter 6, but critics have also indicated that some of this advice may in any case be inappropriate for certain groups in the population because of its financial implications (Lang, 1984), sexist assumptions (Hunt, 1985; Kerr and Charles, 1986), and lack of appreciation of the fact that eating is a social experience (Fieldhouse, 1986).

Anthropologists have long documented how beliefs and practices concerning eating and drinking are affected by many social and cultural factors which may bear little direct relationship to issues of the basic availability and palatability of foodstuffs (Fieldhouse, 1986), far less to concerns about healthy eating. This may be illustrated by considering three aspects of these behaviours: the acceptability of different kinds of food and drink; the meanings behind the sharing of food with others (commensality); and the differing evaluations of the physical end product of eating, i.e. the body size.

Different social groups vary in their ideas about what they think of as food, what foods are appropriate to the ages and circumstances of their members, and the effects of food on people's health generally (Eckstein, 1980). Many Latin American cultures, for example, distinguish between 'hot' and 'cold' foods. This is a complex classification which may not reflect the actual physical properties of the foods themselves (Molony, 1975), and which may also vary between individuals in the same culture. It relates to basic beliefs that health is a temperate condition and that disease results from an imbalance between 'hot' and 'cold'. Foods defined as 'hot' or 'cold' play a major role in avoiding imbalance. Certain groups in society are perceived as particularly susceptible to such imbalances, and special attention is paid to the 'hot' and 'cold' food intake of, for example, women during menstruation, pregnancy and at postpartum. Thus, during menstruation, which is regarded as a 'warm' state, foods defined as 'cold' must be avoided as they may cause cramps. Pregnancy and lactation are also 'warm' states when 'cold' foods may be prohibited. Harwood (1971) found that Puerto Rican women thought pregnancy was a 'hot' state and avoided 'hot' foods and medicines (such as vitamins and iron) since these might cause babies to be born with rashes or red skins.

Similarly, public health programmes aimed at ensuring an uncontaminated water supply through boiling or other means have encountered problems because of basic beliefs and customs surrounding water consumption. For example, studies have shown that even when information about the health implications of boiling contaminated water for drinking has been disseminated at the local level, a variety of cultural factors may result in variation in uptake of the practice. Not the least of these factors is the meaning attached to boiled water itself. For example, people have associated the boiling of water with sickness and may be resistant to carrying out the process if they feel perfectly well. An early study by Wellin (1958) in Peru led him to conclude that:

'To understand fully the varieties of response to the water boiling issue, it was necessary to take into account many sectors of culture, including definitions of health and illness, the organisation of kitchens and the scheduling of daily chores, mobility aspirations, the prevailing status system, and the community's patterns of utilisation of its water resources (p. 18).

Anthropologists have also demonstrated how the way in which food is distributed and shared is expressive of social relationships, of structural differences within groups, and of symbolic and religious values. Food sharing and gift giving may be used to express emotions such as friendship, love, sympathy and marital or familial discord. For example, the Havik Brahmin woman, who marriage separates from close contacts with her female relatives and previous friends, may express her distress over marital and familial discords through manipulation of expectations about food-sharing. (Nichter has called this 'kitchen politics'). She may, for instance, be unattentive to her husband's 'honoured guests' by making them wait for sustenance, and then not providing them with the expected kinds of food and drinks (Nichter, 1981). Food may also be used to assert and acknowledge status differences, most obviously in the commensality taboos of the Hindu caste system, and to celebrate, perhaps by its conspicuous consumption, significant events in the lives of individuals or groups, for example the potlach feasts of the American Indians (Fieldhouse, 1986).

On an everyday level, ideas about domestic cleanliness connected with sharing food and drink may be influenced by social structural norms rather than (if at all) by any theory of germs and contagion. Thus, in some Tunisian villages, family members eat and drink from the same utensils using fingers or shared cutlery. Teitelbaum (1969) showed how decisions about commensality reflected social relationships. The Tunisians felt that close friends and kin would not transmit sickness when sharing food as they should have good feelings for one another. However, enemies, strangers or those of lower social standing might harbour bad feelings which could cause sickness; and eating with such people was best avoided. Thus risks to physical health might occur from dining with the wrong companions.

Finally, attitudes to what constitutes, 'normal' body size have varied historically and cross-culturally. In Havik society, for example, body weight is a frequent topic of conversation, and a reasonable weight gain is associated with emotional well-being. Conversely, loss of weight is seen as an emotional as well as a physical indicator that something is wrong with a woman's life (Nichter, 1981). For Tunisians, plumpness is also valued and is associated with good health and a 'worry-free attitude'. A lack of worries is perceived as reflecting more comfortable economic circumstances which allow people to afford fattening foods such as meat and oil (Teitelbaum, 1969). Anthropological approaches thus reveal social and cultural factors underlying attitudes to body size and suggest the value of applying such analyses to Western cultures. Too frequently 'only physical parameters and consequences are used to judge the value and desirability of eating habits' (Fieldhouse, 1986). By and large, in Western society, plumpness is taken as an indicator that something is or may be 'wrong' with an individual or bodes ill for the future, either emotionally or physically. The treatment and avoidance of obesity is largely based on ideals of preventive medicine. However, as such measures tend not to exist in cultures where overweight is valued, the assessment of obesity as a 'problem' must also be seen as a reflection of the current norms of slimness in Western society (Orbach, 1978).

Studies of Health and Illness in Western Cultures: The Contributions of Social Science

Much of the information available today about health and health behaviours has been gathered indirectly through the study of illness and disease. Nevertheless, over the past two decades, a considerable body of social scientific research has documented the importance of sociological and psychological factors in the development of illness behaviours. Only in recent years has attention broadened to address factors affecting health as well as illness. In addition, awareness of the limitations of studying these behaviours within a biomedical model and, as outlined in the previous section, a growing appreciation of the pluralism of health beliefs and behaviours within Western health systems, has stimulated interest in studying lay (or emic) definitions, and the everyday contexts of health behaviours. Nowadays it is accepted that

> every individual draws on those meanings that are socially available to him (her) to interpret his (her) experience of illness. Thus, whilst an important implication of illness appears to be departure from 'normal', 'standard' or 'average', the meaning of normality with regard to bodily experience varies immensely between individuals and between social groups (Fitzpatrick, 1982, p. 4).

This section will examine some of the main findings of these different branches of research which, taken as a whole, demonstrate the complexities involved in the social construction of health and illness.

In the 1950s an important early contribution was Parsons' development of the concept of the sick role and his analysis of its functional implications for the social system in structuring and controlling the 'deviancy' of illness (Parsons, 1951). Health, in Parsons' view, was fundamentally involved with the functional prerequisites of the social system. For a society to have too low a general level of health or too high a level of illness would be dysfunctional. This stimulated social scientists to examine cultural, structural and, to a lesser extent, interactional variables affecting the development of illness behaviour. However, both the topics chosen for research and the methods employed continued to be dominated by a positivist, biomedically based, approach, which fitted well with the Parsonian functionalist perspective. This approach entailed specifying in advance the variables to be investigated. Moreover, these variables were, in fact, derived from problems considered of relevance by the providers of formal medical care (Idler, 1979). Often studies (explicity or implicitly) were concerned with the basic question of 'compliance', i.e. why certain groups of individuals over-used under-used, misused or did not use available medical services. Not surprisingly reaction to this body of evidence included the critique of the 'medicalization' of society (Zola, 1975) and the analysis of medicine as an agent of social control (Illich, 1975; Navarro, 1976).

Thus, the early work may be criticized for underestimating the power relationships inherent in social definitions of what constitutes health and illness (Freidson, 1970b). It was, however, useful in that it did draw attention to the non-medical factors affecting individual perceptions of illness, the processes of adopting the sick role, and decisions about medical care. Studies of reactions to pain have shown that variations in perception and behaviour occur which cannot be explained in purely biomedical or in psychological terms (Zborowski, 1952; Sternbach and Tursky 1965), as Freidson (1970b) has concluded

> Responses to pain also vary by the ethnic or cultural experience of the group from which the individual has learned what meanings to find in his experience and which provides the individual with continual reinforcement for such meanings. (p. 283)

Variations also occur in the processes of acknowledging to others that one is sick and of taking, or not taking, some action to seek help. Freidson described the interpersonal influences on an individual in the early stages of recognizing signs and symptoms of illness as the 'lay referral system' (Freidson, 1960). The reactions of lay peers to an individual's sickness may be more or less congruent with those of medical professionals, and this, Freidson maintained, affects utilization of formal medical services. In addition, the structure of the relevant lay community varies in its cohesiveness and thus, he suggested, in the strength of the pressures it may exert on the individual. This attempt to relate individual behaviour to its sociological context is valuable theoretically but problematic empirically because of the difficulties in operationalizing concepts such as 'community'. Also, the fact that illnesses/sicknesses vary in their social acceptability means that they will not all be made similarly available for assessment by lay others.

Further non-physiological triggers affecting the decison to seek medical help were suggested by Zola (1973). Basing his theories on a study of new patients of Italian or Irish origin attending an outpatient clinic, he suggested five triggers which had prompted the patients eventually to seek medical help for symptoms which many of them had apparently tolerated for some time. The triggers were (a) an interpersonal crisis (b) the perceived interference of the ailment with social or personal relationships, (c) sanctioning from others wishing the ill person to seek medical help (the lay referral system in action?), (d) perceived interference with vocational or physical activity and (e) the sick person's assessment of the appropriate length of time that symptoms should last before seeking medical help (temporalizing of symptoms).

Zola's work was stimulating in its description of how factors largely beyond the actual experience of sickness can affect the course of action taken by the afflicted individual. As with Freidson's work, however, the definition of exactly who are the relevant 'significant others' exerting pressure on the sick person remains an empirical question (McKinlay, 1975). Also, there is an inherent assumption that symptoms of illness are clearly perceived by the individual and significant others as different from a more usual 'symptom free' state of health. Such an assumption has been challenged theoretically and empirically. Examining the continuous interplay between health and disease from a historical perspective, the microbiologist Dubos (1965) concluded that health was a *modus vivendi* which allowed imperfect men to achieve a rewarding and not too painful existence while they coped with an imperfect world. Empirical studies also support a sceptical view of the existence of any ideal state of disease-free health. When health complaints were studied more broadly in populations it appeared that, in fact, medically presented symptoms were simply the 'tip of an iceberg' of experience of physical ailments (Wadsworth *et al.*, 1973; Hannay, 1979). Thus, studies focusing on processes of seeking formal medical help not only ignore an enormous body of lay health care (Levin *et al.*, 1977), but also present too narrow a definition of the relationship between health and illness (Idler, 1979).

Another approach to understanding the development of illness behaviour and the seeking of formal medical help concentrated on the development of social psychologically oriented models. Two examples are Mechanic's analysis of help seeking in the presence of signs and symptoms and Rosenstock's Health Belief Model which was concerned with preventive health behaviour. The Health Belief Model has been considered in detail in Chapter 1.

Rooted firmly in a functional biomedical perspective, Mechanic (1968) outlined ten variables which affected the individual's perception of and reaction to 'deviant signs and symptoms'. These overlapping variables dealt, for example, with the individual's perception of the seriousness, persistence and implications of the symptoms; different tolerance levels of individuals; the amount of disruption of everyday life and the place assigned to illness in competition with other needs; and the medical, social and cultural information possessed by the individual about the symptoms and potentially available treatments. Mechanic did acknowledge the possibilities of competing definitions of the symptoms: for example that different saliencies might be attached by the patient and the doctor, as well as by the individual and others in his or her environment. However, working within the biomedical model there was always the assumption that illness was dysfunctional and that the 'rational' solution lay within the formal medical system. Not only does this tend to reify the concept of disease and underplay its social construction but, by focusing on individual reactions, it also neglects the possibility that there may have been social causes for the disease (Idler, 1979).

During the 1970s the limitations of researching predominantly biomedically defined illness and treatment began to be appreciated. Surveys indicated that many signs and symptoms of illness were, in fact, never taken to doctors and, increasingly, the role of alternative definitions and lay processes of dealing with illness were documented (Wadsworth et al., 1973; Hannay, 1979 Dunnell and Cartwright, 1972). Various assumptions inherent in adopting a biomedical approach were questioned. Firstly the concentration on service use had implied that medically defined appropriate behaviours were the most rational and acceptable courses of action for all concerned (Dingwall, 1976). Secondly, the claimed 'objectivity' of medical judgments with their appeal to scientific legitimacy was challenged. The assumption in most research had been that such judgements would be more accurate in assessing illness than the 'subjective' statements of patients which drew on much wider spheres of relevance (Freidson, 1976b; MacIntyre, 1976; Hunt et al., 1986). Finally, a large body of research began to detail the problematical nature of actual encounters of patients with health professionals. In particular the unequal power relationship between doctors and patients was highlighted; and the social messages and meanings being communicated in the encounters, many of which were unconnected with the medical purpose at hand, were dissected (Bloor and Horobin, 1974; Stimson and Webb, 1975; Cartwright and Anderson, 1981; Roberts, 1985).

Dissatisfaction with the limitations of biomedically based research was paralleled by the development of the interpretive approach in the social sciences. This offered both a critique of positivist methods and a shift in topics seen as relevant for study. The realities of health and illness, it was claimed, should not be treated as medically defined 'givens', but as dynamic social constructions (Dingwall, 1976; Fabrega, 1974). Health and illness behaviours should be seen as created, recreated and negotiated in the everyday interactions of individuals. (Interactions with the formal health care system may be only one element of such behaviour if, indeed, they actually take place at all.) Drawing on the work of Schutz (1972), the focus of study, it was claimed, should be the subjective meaning of social action. Individuals draw on their social stocks of knowledge and biographical experiences to perceive and interpret the situations, events and experiences they encounter. These interpretations are dynamic and are continuously re-examined and reformulated in the light of interactions with others and the situational context. Thus, illness was now treated as a problematical experience and the individual was analysed as a conscious and reflective actor engaged in the process of making sense of various kinds of bodily changes within the framework of lay knowledge (West, 1979). This appreciation of the sociological complexities of illness behaviour (see Locker

(1981) for a study of the cognitive and interactional processes by which meanings of illness are constructed), and the importance of phenomenological meaning and social context in its development, were some of the reasons why the framework of analysis was broadened to address the study of health as well as that of illness. A further influence on the development of a different approach to studying health and illness came from work, such as that of Douglas (1970), which emphasised the interactive relationship between self, body and society. She stated that,

> The social body constrains the way the physical body is perceived. The physical experience of the body, always modified by the social categories through which it is known, sustains a particular view of society. There is a continual exchange of meanings between the two kinds of bodily experience so that each reinforces the categories of the other. (p. 65)

The issue of the social significance of the human body was also addressed by Manning and Fabrega (1973) when they compared the social construction of illness in Western and traditional societies. They contended that the modern Western view of the body is biologically based and derived from Western medicine and germ theory. The biomedical tradition objectifies the body and tends to separate it from its social and ecological environment. They called this process 'disembodiement' and contrasted it with traditional cultures where a more 'embodied' sense of self often exists. By this they meant that, taking the Mayans of Mexico as an example, illness was experienced as a social event and seen as caused by the Gods. That the Mayans' interpretation of illness reflected human and spiritual relationships is further demonstrated by the healing work of the Shaman, whose main therapeutic aim was to restore the group's cohesiveness and harmony. More recently Crawford has applied this kind of analysis to health in Western cultures and claimed that this is 'a category of experience that reveals tacit assumptions about individuals and social reality' (p. 62). The very taken-for-grantedness of health and its incorporation into 'normal' everyday life means that it is a reflection of basic concerns and conventional understandings in society, most particularly notions of 'well-being' or 'quality of life' (Crawford, 1984).

Thus developments in the social sciences have contributed to a new approach to studying public health which is critical of the dominance of the biomedical model; which stresses the pluralism of concepts of health and illness in Western cultures; and which redirects attention to the importance of sociocultural contexts in understanding behaviour. Moreover, proponents of this approach stress that distinction must be made between the subjective experience of illness and biomedical concepts of disease; and that each set of concepts is developed in particular social structural contexts. This distinction has been described as 'patients suffer illness: physicians diagnose and treat disease' (Eisenberg, 1977, p. 9). It is now appreciated that 'health' and 'being healthy' are themselves problematical concepts which cannot be treated as simply the obverse of illness or disease. In the next section one branch of research reflecting this different approach will be described: that of lay concepts of health and illness.

Lay Concepts of Health and Illness

Many of the conceptual and empirical difficulties in studying health have been addressed in the preceding chapters. Researchers into lay health beliefs in Western cultures have regularly claimed that people find it difficult to talk about positive health (Pill and Stott,

1982, 1985; Blaxter and Paterson, 1982). It has proved easier to gather empirical data about negative health and illness and this is reflected in the content of many studies to date (Cornwell, 1984). Blaxter and Paterson (1982) concluded that their working-class female respondents did not have a concept of positive health. Pill and Stott's sample of Welsh working-class women did express positive conceptions of physical and mental health and well-being. It was claimed, however, that this varied within the sample, with women who were more aware of 'lifestyle factors' and of the possibility of influencing environmental conditions being more likely to have some positive concept of health (Pill and Stott, 1985). One of the explanations for this is that health is a taken-for-granted state whereas illness is a problematical interruption which has to be managed. Indeed, it has been suggested that anthropologically based studies have indicated that phenomena presenting practical problems (such as illness) generate a more complex body of knowledge than those which are seen as non problematical (such as health) (Locker, 1981). Also, as Hunt (1987) has commented: 'The healthy body/ mind does not demand conscious attention and the focus is outward not inward' (p. 6). It could also be suggested that some groups in Western cultures might devalue a preoccupation with a basically 'nonproblematical' state of health as self-indulgence or hypochondria (Cornwell, 1984; Backett, 1987). Thus, it may be argued that apparent difficulties in tapping concepts of positive health empirically may derive from basic problems of meaning. However, as will be discussed in the final section, there are also several methodological reasons why this might be the case.

Much of the literature on lay concepts of health and illness has continued to have a medical focus, albeit within a much broader understanding of social context. It seems that, although phenomenological, structural and sociopsychological concepts have certainly been addressed in the course of the studies, much of the British work has had a biomedical 'problem' as its impetus. More studies have, therefore, been carried out with working-class groups who have a higher level of medically defined ill health, and who are seen as being more problematical than other social groups. Studies have focused on ideas of illness causation and responsibility for health with relevance to preventive medicine (Pill and Stott, 1982); on lay concepts grounded in work and family experience which have implications for service use (Cornwell, 1984); on 'how perceptions of health experiences might in poor socioeconomic circumstances, create attitudes of apathy towards health care and conflict with health professionals, and that these attitudes might be transmitted through generations' (Baxter and Paterson, 1982, p3); on how lay beliefs about health maintenance and illness prevention might explain the uneven impact of health education on working-class and middle-class groups (Calnan, 1985); and on understanding why the illness and help-seeking behaviour of Pathan mothers in the North of England did not reflect the suggested incidence of depression amongst them (Currer, 1986). This is not so obvious in the work of Donovan (1986) and Williams (1983). Donovan examined the perceptions and experiences of health among two groups of people of Asian and Afro-Caribbean descent. Williams work on lay concepts of health among elderly Aberdonians can also be seen as an exception to this but his qualitative analysis was part of a wider programme on ageing which included many questions about physical ailments.

The difficulty with studies having a medical focus is that, although undoubtedly unintentional, the researchers' assessment of those lay concepts relevant to a biomedically defined 'issue' simply leads once again to understanding why certain groups do not behave as they 'ought'. In addition, if one accepts that the realities of health and illness are socially constructed, it becomes evident that these 'oughts' are determined by the current state of knowledge of biomedical science; and that the 'appropriate' health-related behaviours are still expected of the individual, albeit with a greater appreciation of his or her social constraints. Also it must always be recognized that people may be carrying out health-related behaviours for many reasons other than those concerned with health, and it is therefore crucial further to understand these subjective meanings in their own right. For example, an individual may take up a sport for its associated social life, to get out into the fresh air, to escape from domestic commitments or to relieve a guilty conscience about excesses of eating and drinking. In fact Pill (1986) has recently concluded:

> Much more attention needs to be paid to what behaviours people themselves perceive as relevant for health maintenance and claim actually to perform, regardless of their objective effectiveness or approval by the medical establishment. (p. 14)

Studies in France and America seem to have been less restricted in their initial definition of the research problem. They have attempted to 'show that conceptions of health and illness have their own coherency, independently of the categories of medical terminology,' (Pierret, 1986, p. 1). Herzlich (1973), for example, interviewed 80 middle-class respondents and identified a competing tension between their views that *illness* was actively determined by the way of life of modern urban society whereas *health* was internally determined by the individual's constitution, temperament and heredity. Pierret (1986) studied five different socio economic groups and was concerned to see how type of employment and position in the labour market affected and reflected their conceptions of the body and ideas about health and illness. Unlike these two qualitative studies, D'Houtaud and Field (1984, 1986) based their analysis on a survey question about the meaning of health as part of a questionnaire on preventive health care. They concluded that responses were clearly linked to socioeconomic status. The non-manual classes, who could be defined as the managers of social tasks, viewed health in more personalized, positive and expressive terms compared with the manual classes, the performers of the social tasks, who were more alienated from their health and viewed it in more negative and instrumental terms.

In America, Crawford (1984) carried out qualitative interviews with white middle-class women under 40 concerning their thoughts on health. He analysed their views in terms of the relationship between body and society and concluded that the tensions they expressed between health and well-being as 'being in control' or as 'a release from pressures' reflected competing structural mandates for discipline (for example in work) or for pleasure (for example in consumption and leisure). Crawford took an interpretive as well as structural approach to the social construction of health and maintained that

> Dominant cultural notions shape our concepts of health in complex relations with meanings that emerge from concrete physical-emotional-social experiences. These experiences do not simply conform to cultural mandates. The body is not only a symbolic field for the reproduction of dominant values and conceptions; it is also a site for resistance to and transformation of those systems of meanings. (p. 95)

Not only have studies of lay concepts differed in underlying purpose, they have also varied methodologically. Although all of the studies have had an open-ended or semistructured component, they have varied in the number of times respondents have been interviewed, the extent to which there has been flexibility in following up respondents' own constructions, and the readiness to quantify the material either in scales or tables, or to present data thematically. There are nevertheless some important themes which tend to recur. The major contributions of the studies to date have been (a) to begin to document the complexity and variety of lay health concepts within Western cultures; (b) to elucidate some of the non-medical meanings underlying health and illness behaviour and examine the alternative and often contradictory rationales involved; and (c) to demonstrate the importance of the individual's interpretation and situational contexts in generating such meanings. These three areas will now be used as a framework to draw out some of the lay concepts (and sociological constructs) in the current literature.

The complexity and variety of lay concepts of health and illness in Western cultures

There is a growing body of data documenting the lay concepts which exist alongside the dominant body of Western biomedical knowledge. However, these data must be treated as still somewhat preliminary as, with some exceptions, they have tended to reflect 'public accounts' of health and illness. Public accounts are those replies usually given in response to more formal abstract questions about health, such as those of a researcher. Whilst incorporating both medical and commonsense theories these accounts tend to be non-controversial, to reflect normative values and to uphold the social order. In contrast, 'private accounts' are more usually given when the respondent has met the interviewer more than once, are often expressed in the form of personalised stories, and explain individual feelings and behaviours by reference to 'material concerns and practical constraints that intrude into matters of health and illness' (Cornwell, 1984, p. 133).

This finding has important implications for public health as well as for research and the resulting data from which conclusions may be drawn. Most notably it raises questions about the relationship between respondents' accounts and their actual behaviour. Which, if either, of these two sets of retrospective legitimations, the 'public' or the 'private', may be taken as more influential for subsequent actions? Also, the analysis of 'private' accounts indicates a much more complex, often contradictory, and contextually based set of legitimations for health-related behaviours. By contrast, if, as may be argued, survey research tends to elicit 'public' accounts, these would appear to constitute a less dynamic set of legitimations. Moreover, 'public' accounts appear to be characterized by respondents seeking to provide either socially appropriate replies, or those answers which they feel the interviewer requires. For researchers this raises once more the problematical issue of the interactional nature of social research which, as those taking an interpretive approach would suggest, must be more self-consciously appraised in any project. For public health, this argues for the increasing use of multitmethod data bases to inform policy and health educational decision-making.

If it is accepted that 'public accounts' have dominated the research literature to date, it is not surprising that variations in lay concepts of health between different groups of the population, for example between classes, sexes, age or ethnic groups, seem to be more those of degree of emphasis rather than of kind. For example, Williams (1983) found that his elderly Aberdonians of all classes held similar concepts of health to those of Herzlich's middle-class, middle-aged Parisians. Pill and Stott (1982, 1985) also found broadly comparable concepts in their sample of working-class Welsh women). Health was viewed as (a) the absence of illness, (b) as a reserve of strength on which to draw, and (c) as an equilibrium or fit with one's way of life and normal obligations. This third category, which may be interpreted as functional fitness, is a theme which recurs in all of the studies and is not surprising in view of Kelman's (1975) analysis of the fit of functionalist views of health with the demands of a capitalist mode of production in Western society. Blaxter (1983), in fact, found fitness for normal roles to be the main way in which her working-class respondents assessed their health and that of their children. Equally, although Cornwell (1984) identified many sex differences in the knowledge, attitudes and responses to illness of her working-class Londoners, the dominant theme for both sexes was their need to show that they were at all times ready and willing to work, be it inside or outside the home. Health for Asian and Afro-Caribbean respondents was seen as a residual state, particularly of not being ill. Again, the importance of health was linked to functional concerns of home and work; but of interest was their view of a pristine state of health, associated with youth, which became eroded both over time and by the British environment (Donovan, 1986).

The work in this area has undoubtedly begun to reveal the complexity and richness of lay concepts of health and illness. However, much more comparative data grounded in the everyday lives and concerns of different groups in the population are required before firmer conclusions can be drawn about variations between them. Both Calnan and Pill have already cautioned that some apparent variations between classes may be methodological artefacts and simply reflect the greater facility of middle-class groups to express more complex multi dimensional definitions when faced with abstract questions in a formal interview setting (Pill and Stott, 1985; Calnan and Johnson, 1985). Equally, whilst the form of the interview can affect responses so also can the kinds of questions asked. It seems that biographical questions focusing on the individual's personal health experiences have tended to elicit more negative concepts of health than abstract questions which elicited 'public accounts' reflecting socially approved and more positive replies (Calnan and Johnson, 1985). In fact Cornwell (1984) found that the private accounts given by her respondents dealt only with negative concepts or illness and concluded that, people did not spend time recalling periods of their lives in which they knew what it was to feel healthy or talk about feeling well at all' (p. 134).

Subjective meanings and rationales underlying health and illness behaviour

The work on lay concepts has also emphasized the importance of subjective interpretations in understanding health-related behaviours. The embeddedness of concepts of health and illness in all aspects of people's domestic and working lives means that, for them, biomedical interpretations of reality are simply one resource amongst many. Thus, behaviour seen as 'irrational' in biomedical terms may be a perfectly valid response when understood from the viewpoint of the individual, or groups, concerned. The existence of alternative and competing subjective meanings behind health-related behaviours is crucial to any realistic appraisal of public health.

There are many examples of this in the literature. Fatalism or a lack of feeling of control over health and illness may, in fact, accurately reflect an individual's personal experience of powerlessness to affect the social and political forces shaping her life (Pill and Stott, 1985; Blaxter and Paterson, 1982; Askham, 1975). For example, Pill's respondents (like Herzlich's) perceived their own way of life as inherently unhealthy and stressed the importance of the genetic constitution and environmental factors as influencing their susceptibility to ill health. Pill (1985) therefore concluded that the women in her sample:

> accorded a relatively low priority to individual action in the genesis of illness causation and they may be closer to the truth than many of the more simplistic messages of health educators would have them believe. (p. 988)

Moreover, subjective interpretations affect the place accorded to a concern for good health in people's lives. If everyday life is viewed as involving competing demands, strains and priorities, concern for health must be treated as problematical; it may not be the most salient or pressing priority (Backett, 1987). In addition, individuals may be carrying out wide ranges of behaviours which they view as health protective, but which may not be medically legitimated and have little connection with formal medical care (Harris and Guten, 1979). Even if individuals are carrying out 'healthy behaviours' this may also be for reasons other than maintaining or protecting their health (Anderson, 1983). Moreover, study of alternative subjective rationales has increased our understanding of behaviour considered medically 'unhealthy'. Graham (1986), for instance, has argued that many socially deprived young mothers may use cigarette smoking as a means of structuring their day, and to give themselves psychological space for a self-directed activity without abdicating the demands of child care.

Studies such as those described above have revealed some of the subjective and sociocultural meanings behind health-related behaviours. They have also begun to indicate that many incompatibilities and inconsistencies can coexist in people's systems of subjective meanings about health. For example, Cornwell's respondents saw inequalities in health as a product of nature, but at the same time held individuals responsible for their place in the hierarchy (Cornwell, 1984). Dissecting phenomenological meanings has, moreover, allowed researchers to begin to differentiate between concepts which may previously have been placed on a single dimension. Calnan (1985) found that, for his respondendents, promoting health and preventing disease were not direct opposites and that both middle and working-class women had much clearer knowledge about the former than the latter. Another example was that whilst the women appreciated the positive benefits of taking regular exercise in terms of well-being or feeling fitter, this did not mean that they saw lack of regular exercise as necessarily harmful to their health. Even amongst well educated and informed social groups, there may very well be a conceptual gap between understanding the claimed scientific links between behaviours and health, and sustaining the belief that preventive health behaviour will actually reap positive results. They, like other groups, may still find it easier to opt for short term rewards rather than long term pay offs (Backett, 1987). Thus, one contribution to public health of many of these explorations of subjective meanings is that they facilitate understanding of the well-known gap between knowledge and behaviour in relation to health and illness.

The importance of interpretations of sociocultural, biographical, and social-situational contexts for understanding health related behaviours

Perhaps the most recurrent theme of all emerging from the study of lay concepts is that of health and illness as moral constructs. Responsibility, blame, guilt, hypochondria and stoicism are just a few of the morally evaluative terms regularly used by respondents when considering these matters. As has been previously indicated, anthropological studies have shown the importance of the spiritual and moral significance of illness in non-Western societies. Applying this kind of analysis to Western medicine, Young (1982) concluded that a major feature of the power of physicians was that they exculpate the sick person by taking on the social accountability for his or her behaviour. The demonstration of the presence of such evaluative systems alongside the supposedly objective directives of Western medicine has been an important contribution of those taking an interpretive or ethnographic approach.

Moral evaluations affect how people talk about health and illness and what they choose to tell a researcher. Herzlich (1973) outlined different interpretations which affected an individual's response to illness. Her respondents described illness as an 'occupation', requiring the individual to fight and control it; as a 'destroyer', which meant that the inactivity as a consequence of illness was deplored, and the best strategy was seen as avoiding or ignoring it; and as a 'liberator', which meant that illness was perceived as freeing the individual from his or her everyday commitments. Moral evaluations of claims to illness also mean that the individual's motivations may be called into question. Thus, an individual may be judged as demonstrating an unwillingness to face up to normal life; as using claims to illness to deal with other disorders; or as using illness as a means of achieving other gains (Locker, 1981). If a claim or response to illness is not regarded as legitimate, the individual may be subjected to moral scrutiny, judgement and pressure.

The work of Cornwell (1984) usefully linked concepts of responsibility for illness to work and sex roles. She found that, in 'public' accounts, good health was perceived as, 'a reward for a good life, meaning a life of moderation and virtue, cleanliness and decency, and above all, a life of hard work' (p. 128). Also, it was important to demonstrate the 'right attitude' to health, and the moral prescription for a healthy life was a cheerful stoicism. Moreover, it was important to demonstrate that illness was 'real', preferably medically legitimated, and, ideally, something for which an individual was not personally responsible or did not just 'give in to'.

Cornwell identified sex differences in how her respondents described their reactions to feeling unwell. She related these directly to the sexual division of labour. Accounts indicated that the men apparently had no qualms about giving in to symptoms at home, and expected the women to look after them so that they would be fit enough to try to 'work it off' the next day. The women, however, were resentful of this behaviour. Their response to symptoms was just to 'carry on', but also to cut down on their domestic obligations so that they would not have to give up altogether. Cornwell's analysis highlighted the importance of considering subjective meanings behind the concept of health as functional ability. Men and women held a similar perspective on the moral significance of work but the actual nature of their work and their relationship to it varied between the sexes. This affected how they perceived functional constraints when they felt unwell.

The data on moral evaluations of good health tend to be much more sparse. On a general level researchers have criticized the shift of emphasis of responsibility for good health from society to the individual as 'victim-blaming' (Crawford, 1977). Studies have indicated that the way in which an individual perceives choices affecting health may involve a different set of experiential priorities from those of medical experts or politicians. For example, the adoption of individual responsibility for preventive health practices may seem both irrelevant and unattainable to a working-class person faced with limited resources, poverty and daily crises (Pill and Stott, 1985; Cornwell, 1984). Whilst an economically secure middle-class person may find it easier to accept the concept of individual responsibility for health, he or she may still experience confusion and guilt about perceived inabilities to incorporate the socially approved health practices into everyday life (Crawford, 1984; Backett, 1987).

Thus, the current fashion for maintaining or promoting one's own good health attracts varied, and often contradictory, lay evaluations. Studies indicate that being overly concerned with one's health may be as open to criticism as is its neglect (Cornwell, 1984). Moreover there seems to be a social pressure to claim good health, since its opposite may imply failure or blame. For example, women may be unlikely to describe their families as unhealthy since this could be construed as a reflection on their competence as mothers and carers (Blaxter and Paterson, 1982; Graham, 1982). Whilst health may be a central value in Western societies it does not have the same meaning or moral imperative for everyone.

An interpretive approach also acknowledges the salience of an individual's biographical experience for making sense of signs and stimuli in everyday life. This must have particular potency when the problematical situation involves the individual's own body. Western biomedical knowledge entails abstraction and generalization about the body, but for each individual, health and illness remain unique experiences. Studies of lay concepts indicate that the individual regularly uses biographical knowledge, whether related to physical or social experience, as a resource to make sense of health and illness. Individuals with a higher level of education seem, however, often better able to present their experiences in a more abstract framework (Pill and Stott, 1985; Calnan and Johnson, 1985). Nevertheless, it has yet to be demonstrated that there is a relationship between the lay articulation of a more 'scientific' appraisal of health and illness and its translation into actual behaviour. Biographical factors could still be the more significant motivational forces. It has been found that the most common criteria for assessing vulnerability are previous or current experiences of an illness or its signs and symptoms (Calnan and Johnson, 1985). Helman (1978) found biographical experience to be important in folk models of infection concerning cold, chills, and fevers. Lay concepts related the aetiology of such complaints to ideas about the relationship between individuals and their experience of 'cold forces' in the environment; to behavioural factors such as making oneself vulnerable to cold; and to the risk of infection inherent in any social relationship. Some of these folk theories contradicted the biomedical model, yet Helman suggested that, for various reasons, the everyday 'operational model' of diagnosis and treatment used by GPs was in fact often closer to the folk model.

It is worth repeating that different kinds of questions elicit different responses and that the vast majority of studies have asked questions which elicit a more generalized 'public' response. When respondents have become more familiar with a researcher and are asked to describe their own personal health a different range of interpretations are put forward with a much greater emphasis on biographical factors (Cornwell, 1984). Such biographical information provides crucial contextual meaning which illuminates lay accounts of health and illness. Moreover, an individual's biography is also used by others in assessment, for, as Locker (1981) has pointed out:

> Health is a master status ascribed on the basis of certain features of an individual's biography and is independent of their state at any point in time. [Thus, for example] 'He never complains' is a statement about a biography and not a statement about the here and now. Moreover, that biography is not necessarily modified by particular instances where the statement does not apply. (p. 99)

At perhaps the most micro level of all, it is important to consider the influence of individuals' interpretations of social situational contexts on the construction of health and illness behaviour. To date, the main way in which researchers have conceptualized the links between individuals and their social environments has been in terms of 'life style'. In the present state of knowledge, however, it may be more profitable to examine the components making up this somewhat nebulous concept. It is not enough to know that marital status, sex or occupation are statistically associated with different patterns of health and illness. The task now facing health researchers is to begin to understand how individuals given such designations describe their influence on life and health, as mediated through everyday social contexts and situations. Study of individuals' domestic lives may reveal many taken-for-granted assumptions and experiences which affect and reflect aspects of health and illness. As Graham (1984) has pointed out:

> In reality, health attitudes are embedded in domestic activities and these activities – shopping, cooking, washing, watching, waiting – are moulded by the practical constraints of time, space and money. (p. 153)

If it is accepted that reality is socially constructed, it is also valuable to examine the basic interactional processes involved. Dingwall (1976) has pointed out that the mutual monitoring of health status is an important factor in the general mutual monitoring of interactional competence in any social interaction. The focus on illness has meant that more work has been carried out on how individuals interact in professional medical settings than in their everyday lives. Cunningham-Burley (1984) attempted to break away from this when she examined the cultural context of childhood illness. She described some of the sociocultural, biographical and interactional interpretations used by young mothers in the process of making sense of situations when their children were ill.

Alonzo (1979) has made a valuable start by dissecting some interactional processes of everyday illness behaviour. He argued that, since it was now recognized that medically reported illness was only the 'tip of the iceberg', this might suggest that illness or some kind of health status deviation was an everyday, typical experience. Given this, he proposed that:

> the focal issue is whether or not the individual can handle or manage health status deviations and remain within the situation and whether socially defined situations can be ongoing while one (or more) of its participants is symptomatic. (p. 397)

Alonzo examined a variety of situations in which individuals coped with medically unreported health status deviations, and suggested some of the interactional processes whereby illness emerged, was acknowledged, and was then 'contained' in everyday life. He argued that most situations have 'bodily performance expectancies' (p.399) of the physical or mental skills and capacities of their participants. Moreover, following Goffman (1963), he pointed out that situations vary in the strength of role obligations and degree of direct involvement required of participants. This will affect the amount of attention which an individual might legitimately be able to give to any bodily symptoms.

Applying Alonzo's ideas to public health it is evident that work situations, notably manual versus non-manual occupations, will vary in the extent to which certain physical symptoms may be 'contained'. Therefore the amount of clinical morbidity which is subsequently 'allowed' to surface will also vary.

Conclusions

Study of lay concepts provides essential information for understanding the social construction of health and illness. By focusing on unfamiliar societies anthropologists have a long tradition of demonstrating the relevance for behaviour of emic concepts of health. They have also shown the embeddedness of these concepts in many areas of everyday social life, some of which are not directly health-related. Studies cited in this chapter have begun to illuminate such issues in Western societies, and to document the pluralistic nature of health systems despite the dominance of a biomedical model. Such findings have important implications for public health. These concluding remarks will, however, be addressed to some of the methodological and theoretical problems characterizing this emerging area of research. Methodologically, the most challenging problem remains that of how to apprehend concepts of health (rather than just those of illness). It has proved easier for researchers to gain access to concepts of illness, perhaps because illness is usually a problematical state which disrupts and calls into question the flow of everyday life. Good health is a more taken-for-granted state, which perhaps makes its articulation more difficult. Moreover, there may be other sociocultural barriers affecting the ability of respondents to talk about health: for example it may simply be less salient to different groups in society, or an over-preoccupation with one's health may be socially denigrated. If health is a concept which respondents find difficult or inappropriate to verbalize, researchers and those interested in public health must examine why this should be the case.

Problems of gaining access to concepts of health may stem, however, as much from the research approach as from respondent reticence. Often researchers have begun with a biomedically defined problem, or a set of medically approved health-related behaviours, and explored lay concepts as they related to such issues. Moreover, sometimes lay concepts have then been explored in one-off interviews which tend to elicit static, socially approved accounts. There is, perhaps, only so much a respondent feels that he or she 'knows', or perceives as being 'relevant', when questioning is constrained in this way. In the present state of knowledge there is good case for allowing respondents themselves to set the research agenda concerning what is important for their health and how they might achieve it as individuals or in groups. Additionally, it would be useful to investigate how such concepts emerge and affect the various social contexts which make up 'life styles' – such as home, work and leisure. It may well be that the factors individuals perceive as promoting or impeding health bear little relationship to biomedically defined rationality. Methods which allow individuals to describe the complexities of their lives, with an appreciation of change over time, will begin to allow documentation of health behaviour in context.

Much work also remains to be done in the area of theory. Perhaps most importantly, it is necessary to break free of assumptions derived from the biomedical model, many of which continue implicitly in much research design. There are many problems in developing a socially based, salutogenic approach, not the least of which is convincing funding bodies of its worth. Related to this main problem is the development of an approach which is sufficiently flexible to suspend biomedically defined ideas of rationality and explore the alternative rationalities employed by people in their everyday lives. As phenomenologists have pointed out, people draw on many areas of meaning to make sense of their lives, and these meanings may be internally inconsistent and vary over time. Also, in terms of health-related behaviours, it is crucial to appreciate that the most salient factors may originate in areas of people's lives which, at first sight, do not appear directly connected.

Previous research has frequently been too ready to identify specific health-related behaviours and study them detached from the social psychological contexts in which they operate. A greater focus on interactional and social situational constraints and processes would illuminate understanding of their saliency for the individuals involved. Crawford (1984) has pointed out that people often describe their health as variable rather than fixed, and think of it as a state of being that shifts with experience. This argues for the importance of studying both how individuals relate to the situation at hand, and also for investigating respondents' own markers of time changes as well as the sociological constructs of life span.

It is also of interest to note that whilst demographic attributes such as age and sex may be regularly statistically associated with aspects of health and illness, few studies have addressed directly the social processes which lie behind such associations. Moreover, the complexity and dynamism of the social expression of these concepts has been missing from many analyses. Verbrugge (1985) has, for example, pointed out that, 'Once seen as fixed and therefore unremarkable by scientists, age differences are now thought to be more changeable across time as birth cohorts vary more in their attitudes and life experiences' (p. 177).

Sex differences are a particularly neglected area. Statistical evidence clearly shows that women experience higher levels of morbidity and live longer, whereas men suffer more from life-threatening diseases and die earlier (Verbrugge, 1985). These data are the end-product of different sex roles, stresses and life styles yet few researchers have been concerned to make detailed study of the implications for health of the everyday social experiences of men and women (Graham, 1984).

Also of importance is a greater appreciation of the effects of gender on the social production of data about health and illness. This applies to both medical and social scientific data. It has been well documented that the experiences of women may not be accurately perceived or interpreted by a male-dominated medical professions (Roberts, 1985; Graham and Oakley, 1981). Furthermore, medical diagnosis and treatment, which provide baseline statistical data, are affected by physicians' own models of appropriate sex role behaviour (Fisher and Groce, 1985). The role of social scientists is also questionable. Many studies have used women as respondents to gather information about health and illness, and sometimes this information is subsequently generalized to both sexes. Arguably, by treating female and male accounts as interchangeable, and thus ignoring the powerful role of gender in the social construction of knowledge, this may have resulted in quite inaccurate understandingof the reasons behind health and illness behaviours. Many of the major health problems, such as coronary heart disease, are primarily male problems, but the vast majority of survey respondents providing information about it have been women. Much less work has been done on chronic conditions such as arthrosis, which are mainly female. Any change in public health must take account of the different experiences of women and men in society.

Finally, researchers must not shy away from including unmeasurable concepts in the conundrum of health. The time has come to acknowledge that if respondents tell us that peace of mind, love and happiness affect their health then we must accord these the status they deserve.

This chapter has demonstrated the importance of sociocultural factors in the development of health and illness behaviours. The meanings and interpretations underlying behaviours have been shown to be crucial. An area of social life where such meanings may be powerfully constructed and disseminated at the macro level is that of the media. The role of the media is the topic of the next chapter.

CHAPTER 4

The Mass Media: Health Information and its Influence

This chapter examines the images of health and the health information provided by the media, in particular the press and television, and it investigates the role the media might play in promoting health. It also considers the contribution that the media may make to the construction of lay perceptions of health and illness. The media permeate everyday life, reaching the majority of the population by one or several of their modes of communication. The media do not simply entertain, although they do provide many individuals with their dominant leisure activity, but by virtue of attracting such large audiences the mass media are a primary source of information and influence regarding public understanding of social and political structures and processes. The media provide a source of meanings by using particular imagery and interpretive frameworks, and the public can draw on these representations of reality in order to make sense of the society in which they live.

It would be naïve and misguided to assume that audiences are passive receivers of media messages. This is reassuring in the sense that it means they cannot easily be duped or manipulated, but it has serious implications for the success of any campaign which employs the mass media and, at least partially, explains the lack of success of health education programmes aimed at mass audiences. People actively interpret what they see and hear; they select, reject, make judgements and discuss issues raised by the media. Changes in attitudes and behaviour if they do occur are likely to do so only after a period of resistance and contemplation. Thus, it is always difficult to attribute them solely to the media.

This chapter discusses models which have been developed to explain the ways in which the media operate, and the processes involved in news production. This provides the background for the main body of the chapter which focuses on media presentation of health. The coverage that is given to health and health-related issues and the forces which constrain the selection of particular events for reporting and the way in which they are presented are examined. Images of health and the explanation of factors supposed to influence the public health promulgated by the media are discussed. Media effects, and specifically, effects on health-related behaviour and health, are investigated.

Models of the Media

Although the news presented by the press and in television broadcasts is undoubtedly some sort of representation of events occurring in the real world, not everything that is happening becomes news. A variety of constraints, some of which are bureaucratic, others of which are ideational, are operating which force the journalist into the selection of certain events or issues and the rejection of others. It is important to consider the incidents and affairs which are not being given media attention as well as those that are, since public debate about a particular issue is often stimulated by media coverage, and if neglected by the media some issues may never reach the public eye.

The particular constraints that are operating and their relative importance to the eventual media output have been discussed in the literature. A number of models have been proposed which differ with respect to which forces they believe to be the most powerful in shaping news and other media output. The two earliest models described in Cohen and Young (1976) were the mass-manipulative model and the *laissez-faire/commercial* model. In the latter the idea is that news is supplied in response to the demands of the audience. The audience's interests and preferences are catered for, this being essential for attracting the advertising revenue necessary for survival. News is presented in a style which suits the audience. This *laissez-faire* model is generally favoured by journalists themselves because their role is characterized as being more benign than in the mass-manipulative model where news is seen as being 'manufactured' to serve commercial and/or political interests. Here the audience is considered to have a passive role, uncritically soaking up all that the media present and thus being manipulated through acceptance of the view of the world being offered.

These models represent two rather extreme viewpoints. However, elements of each are plausible and may be found in a more recent explanatory model from the cognitive school of thought. In this formulation the journalist is not seen as intentionally biasing or distorting facts, but rather as interpreting and selecting events to fit pre-existing categories which are consistent with his or her view of social reality (Cohen and Young, 1976). The possibility of some commercial bias is not ruled out in this model but it would not be seen as an extreme form of censorship.

The fourth model, from the cognitive-ideological school, takes the previous formulation further and proposes that the interpretive frameworks employed by the media reflect the society's dominant political ideology (Murdoch, 1974). This meaning system is provided by the groups in society which occupy positions of most power. They tend to have greatest access to the media and so their particular explanations and constructions of the social and political situation become promulgated as the accepted ones.

It is not the intention of this discussion to come down in favour of one model over another, indeed the models share certain elements. However, the journalist must use some sort of interpretive framework both for the selection of items and in finding a way to present them. The precise balance of forces that shape the framework will depend partly on the journalist's own ideology but probably even more so on the prevailing politicoeconomic climate.

Issues or events that become news, or feature in some other form of media output, such as television documentary programmes, newspaper editorials or features, magazine articles, or radio magazine programmes, are selected from a myriad of daily happenings and current affairs. Events are often selected as being newsworthy on the basis of their consonance with pre-existing images (Best *et al.*, 1977), these images having been moulded by the particular interpretive frameworks adhered to by the media. News therefore tends to reiterate earlier statements and viewpoints.

Bureacratic/operational constraints that act on the selection procedure arise from the fact that newspapers, news bulletins and, to a lesser extent, other media output are inextricably tied to time. The events that tend to be given news coverage are those that fit in with the 24-hour cycle (Murdoch, 1974). This means that processes of a more long-term nature tend to be ignored or reported in such a way as to make them appear ephemeral. Underlying causes are neglected in preference to the more immediate questions of who did what, where.

Although the focus of the discussion in this section is on news, the same arguments apply to other forms of media output. The presentation of news has to be done in such a way as to be readily assimilated by the audience; therefore, the meanings and imagery used must be widely available and easily understood (Murdoch, 1974). Obviously, this can lead to stagnation in that the public come to regard issues that have been repeatedly presented to them with the same interpretive framework as being 'fact', rather than simply one version of reality with all its inherent biases.

Media Coverage of Health Issues

Coverage of health and health-related issues is found in the press, on television and radio and in magazines. This discussion will focus mainly on health coverage by the dominant media, press and television. This is not to say that magazines, and in particular, women's magazines (Amos, 1984), and radio are not important sources of health information, but other than Amos's work very little research has been directed to assess health coverage by these media.

Press coverage of health-related topics comes in three main forms, news, features/special reports and advice columns. Health appears in a wide variety of television programmes, in news items, in documentary programmes, and in educational/advice programmes, often in magazine style. Television has another type of programme which has no real counterpart in newspapers, namely drama with a health-related theme or health-related component. Of all forms of drama, it is 'soap opera' whose health content has attracted most attention and analysis in the medical and health education literature (Piepe *et al.*, 1986; Lock, 1986; Shaw, 1986; Platt, 1987).

Press coverage of health-related issues has been the subject of a number of detailed studies (Read and Pease, 1971; Best *et al.*, 1977; Combs and Slovic, 1979; Kristiansen, 1983; Kristiansen and Harding, 1984; Wellings, 1985; Harding, 1985; Currie, 1987; Kristiansen and Harding, 1988). However, although critiques of individual television programmes have been written (Anon, 1980a; Anon, 1980b; Bradley and Brooman, 1980; Kennedy, 1980; Adler, 1981; Jenkins, 1983; Turton, 1983), and a content analysis of medical programmes on BBC television has been carried out (Garland, 1984), a systematic analysis of television coverage of health and health-related issues is lacking.

The first problem encountered in any study of media health coverage is definitional. Each time research of this kind is carried out the researcher has to decide which issues are to be categorized as health-related (Kristiansen and Harding, 1984; Garland, 1984) and, depending on that researcher's particular interests and perspectives, so the list of topics selected will vary. This is not a minor point for although most researchers would include any media output concerned with disease or curative medicine, not all would consider that such issues as, for example, damp housing should be included, yet there is good evidence that damp housing is a contributory factor to respiratory illness in children and affects the mental health of adults (Martin *et al.*, 1987). In any case, until what are considered to be health-related issues are more globally agreed upon it will be necessary for researchers to define their terms as they do in the studies described below. In a study of health coverage by the British press, Kristiansen and Harding (1984, 1988) used thirteen topic categories when analyzing the subject matter of articles. Some of these were obviously medically oriented – e.g. medical advances or research, diseases or ailments – and others were less directly related to illness and its treatment such as class inequalities, environmental pollution and traffic safety. In a content analysis of BBC television medical programmes Garland (1984) examined the extent to which the broadcasts reflected the realities and complexities of public health and medical provision. She therefore scored programmes according to whether they covered topics ranging from medical technology and scientific advance to housing and poverty and social status. The findings of both these studies are discussed later.

In an analysis of the content of seven British daily newspapers during July and August 1981, Kristiansen and Harding (1984, 1988) found 1397 articles on health issues; some articles (n=589), however, covered more than one topic so that in total 1986 topics were addressed by the 1397 articles. The percentage of articles covering each topic was as follows: obstetrics (4%); prevention. e.g. seatbelts, health education (15%); medical advances and research (14%); diseases (34%); environmental influences on health, e.g. pollution, working and housing conditions (13%); birth control (5%); addiction or issues of self-control (5%); National Health Services e.g. strikes, funding (13%); medical incompetence (9%); death or euthanasia (11%); disabilities (12%); class inequalities (0.3%); other topics, not defined by the authors (8%).

Of all the health topics it was diseases that clearly received the greatest press attention; and it is striking that they received more than twice as much coverage as issues relating to prevention. A strong disease orientation was also found in a study of the Scottish and UK press 4 years later, in 1985 (Currie, 1987). In this study, which used the same categories of health topics as Kristiansen and Harding, out of a total of 1197 health-related articles there were 74 on AIDS and 100 on cancer. These diseases alone therefore appeared in 15% of the articles. A major difference in the two studies was that drug abuse was found to be receiving considerably greater attention in the more recent study (Currie, 1987); there were 147 articles on drug abuse, which represented 12% of all health-related articles. In the earlier study only 5% of articles covered addictions and problems of self-control which, in addition to drug abuse, included alcohol abuse, smoking and eating disorders. The growth of press interest in drug abuse seemed to mirror the growth of the problem and may have even magnified it, no doubt encouraged by the chances for many an attention-seeking headline, e.g. 'Boy, 14 waits for death in drug city' (*Daily Mail*, July 31, 1985).

It may seem from the example of drug abuse coverage that the press seeks to inform the public about issues of importance and relevance to their health. However, a closer examination of press attention to particular health issues reveals that there is little evidence that the press is a benign adviser on health risks. Indeed, the press has been charged with hindering health by detracting attention from the major causes of ill health and emphasizing instead dramatic and sudden illnesses which are less common (Budd and McCron, 1981). There is no correspondence between the British press's coverage of particular diseases and the mortality statistics for these diseases (Kristiansen, 1983). So, for example, rabies, which caused 1 death in 1980, received attention in 41 articles, but respiratory disease accounting for over 83 000 deaths annually was the subject of only 8 articles.

There is little evidence, therefore, that the press is bringing to the attention of its readership matters that are likely to have most impact on their health. However, a closer analysis of treatment of health issues by different types of press, described below, reveals that different sectors of the population may be being better served by the newspapers that they read than others.

In Garland's (1984) content analysis of television medical programmes there was a heavy bias towards technology, the hospital and the doctor. The 'doctor as communicator' appeared in 94% of programmes and the hospital setting featured in 75%; drug technology and machine technology featured in 58% and 53% of programmes respectively. This was in stark contrast to issues of the family, the environment, housing, poverty, social status and preventive care which together only featured in just over 8% of programmes. The dominant image of medicine portrayed by these broadcasts was that it is expert-dependent, hospital-based and technologically oriented.

The 'Quality' and 'Popular' Press in Britain

Newspapers in Britain may be divided into the 'quality' press, such as *The Times* and the *Guardian,* and the 'popular' press, such as the *Daily Mail* and the *Daily Express.* This classification is used by those who are involved with producing newspapers and those who study the press (McQuail, 1976) and yet it is difficult to find any scientific justification for using such value laden terms, or for assigning particular newspapers to one or other group. The terms were presumably born of the press world and have fallen into common usage. Academics have, perhaps somewhat uncritically, picked up the quality/popular division as a heuristic device to compare the newspapers read by the middle and working classes.

The Joint Committee for National Readership Surveys (JICNARS) gives a profile of the readership of each of Britain's national and regional newspapers. Tables shows the readerships of the main Scottish national and UK national papers in 1985. It reveals the very small percentages of socioeconomic groups IIIb, IV and V that read the quality press.

The quality press and the popular press differ both in their content and their style (Williams, 1966; Smith, 1974; McQuail, 1976). In particular, the quality newspapers have been found to devote more editorial space to coverage of political matters (Seymour-Ure, 1968), and their style has been characterized by greater overall size, fewer pictures and less space given to headlines (McQuail, 1976). More recent studies (Kristiansen and Harding, 1988; Currie, 1987) suggest that the quality and popular newspapers also differ in their coverage of health issues. Using the same classification scheme to categorize health articles, both studies found that the quality press published a significantly greater number of articles on health than the popular press. For example,

Table 4.1
Readership of UK and Scottish National Newspapers

Newspaper	Readership (000s)	I	II	% of Socioeconomic group IIIa	IIIb	IV	V
Popular							
Sun	11717	5	10	20	35	38	26
Mirror	9952	7	10	18	29	31	20
Mail	5021	18	16	15	10	8	6
Express	4910	12	13	15	11	9	7
Star	4374	2	3	6	13	16	10
Record	2010	2	3	5	7	5	
Quality							
Telegraph	2798	29	17	8	2	2	1
Guardian	1435	7	9	5	1	1	1
The Times	1245	17	8	3	1	1	<1
Glasgow Herald	398	4	2	1	<1	<1	<1
Scotsman	240	2	2	1	<1	<1	<1

during the month of July 1985, five quality newspapers were found to feature a mean of 121 health articles and seven popular newspapers carried a mean of only 84 articles (Currie, 1987). Similarly, in 1981 Kristiansen and Harding (1988) found a mean monthly coverage of 144 articles in the quality press and 66 in the popular press. The *Sun*, which attracts the greatest readership from socioeconomic groups IIIb, IV and V, had the poorest coverage of health issues with a monthly average of only 59 articles.

Employing a number of measures to compare press interest in health issues, Kristiansen and Harding (1988) found that there are other important differences between the quality press and the popular press. These are summarized in Table 4.2. The Budd Attention Score which appears in the table is a composite measure incorporating headline size, length of article, page placement and location of the article within the paper. It is believed to yield a more accurate assessment of press interest in a subject than length of article or any one of the other measures alone (Budd, 1964: Kristiansen and Harding, 1974, 1988). The quality press not only gave a higher profile to heath issues, it published a proportionally greater number of articles which were educational in style. It used more reliable sources of information, citing academic journals, books and government reports. The health articles appearing in the quality press were of a more informative nature. In terms of health content, it was found that although curative medicine received more attention from the quality press, greater coverage was also given to social factors in ill health such as unemployment and class inequalities.

Before discussing the wider implications of these differences in terms of variation in health information being supplied to different sectors of society, the press coverage of AIDS by the two types of press is examined in some depth. This particular issue is

Table 4.2
Comparison of Health Coverage By Quality (Q) and Popular (P) Press
(From Kristiansen and Harding, 1988)

Measurement		Comparison of Q and P
Absolute and relative size of articles		Q > P
Use of photographs and diagrams		Q > P
Proportion of articles primarily concerned with health		Q > P
Articles located nearer front of paper		Q > P
Budd Attention Scores		Q > P
Sections of paper where article appears:	home news	Q > P
	overseas news	Q > P
	letters	Q > P
	entertainment	Q < P
	women's	Q < P
	unspecified	Q < P

selected because of the current degree of concern about the spread of the disease in the population and the importance of behaviour in relation to its control.

Content of articles: case study of AIDS

In 1985 AIDS was not yet being considered a major threat to the public health in Britain. Press interest was sporadic. In July of that year a study of the Scottish and UK press (Currie, 1987) revealed that the quality and popular press differed significantly in the newsplay they devoted to AIDS. That month the Hollywood screen star, Rock Hudson, was discovered by the media to be suffering from the 'Killer disease' (*Press and Journal*, 26 July, 1985). Until the first mention of his illness, 'Friends concerned for star Rock' (*Edinburgh Evening News* 23 July 1985), when indeed it was not yet publicized that he had AIDS, there was virtually no coverage being given to AIDS in the popular press (Currie, 1987). Table 4.3 gives details of AIDS coverage in the two types of press in 'pre-' and 'post-Hudson' periods i.e. before and after the first reference to his having AIDS.

Table 4.3
Press Coverage of AIDS

	Total Number of Articles	
	Quality press (n=5)	Popular press (n=7)
1–22 July: pre-Hudson	10	3
23–31 July: post-Hudson	16	29

The table illustrates the dramatic increase in the popular newspapers' interest in AIDS after 'The Anguish of Rock' *Daily Express*, 25 July, 1985, was discovered.

Although the quality press also devoted greater attention to the disease 'post-Hudson', the increase in interest was less marked. These observations seem to lend support to the generally held opinion that the press (and especially the popular press) has an insatiable appetite for the sensational (Lock, 1986).

To be fair, it could be contended that the popular newspapers were employing the well-used vehicle of the personal story for the purpose of educating their readership about the disease; knowing that Hudson's name would attract attention they could then supply useful information to their 'captured' audience. However, a content analysis of the AIDS articles in the quality and popular newspapers lends little support to such speculation.

Using Kristiansen and Harding's (1988) method for analyzing the content of articles about diseases, Currie (1987) evaluated articles on AIDS along nine dimensions: whether there was mention (a) of cause, (b) symptoms (c) treatment, and its success or otherwise, (d) prognosis, (e) prevention, (f) mortality and morbidity statistics (g) the organic process of the illness (h) the subjective experience of the illness and (i) the effect of the illness on daily life. The percentages of articles in each of the quality newspapers and the popular newspapers that mentioned each of the items are presented in Table 4.4.

Table 4.4
Content Analysis of AIDS Articles

	Percentage of articles in	
	Quality press	Popular press
Mention of:		
Cause	40	33
Symptoms	12	37
Treatment	39	18
Prognosis	45	56
Prevention	25	13
Mortality statistics	25	0
Morbidity statistics	17	0
Organic process of illness	4	17
Subjective experience of illness	8	12
Effect of illness on daily life	0	0

The figures in Table 4.4 were generated from a relatively small number of articles, 26 in the quality press and 32 in the popular press, and therefore findings should be treated with some caution. Nevertheless, the differences in content of articles between the two types of paper seem to bear out Kristiansen and Harding's (1988) finding that health coverage in the popular press is less educational. Table 4.4 shows that on those items that would provide readers with potentially useful information with regard to protecting themselves from contracting the AIDS virus, namely, information on causes, prevention, morbidity and mortality statistics, and treatment (or rather the lack of any effective one), the quality press articles gave more coverage. The popular press paid more attention to symptoms which were so unspecific as to be, at best, useless and at worst worrying. They also made more reference to the fatal nature of the disease and the organic process of the illness. By concentrating on these aspects of AIDS, the popular press seemed to be using Hudson's plight to entertain rather than to educate. As Dorkins (1986) pointed out, 'medicine as entertainment is an area which certainly has not escaped the attention of the media' (p. 3), and human interest stories occupy a substantial proportion of editorial space, especially in the popular press (Curran and Seaton, 1985).

The sensational style of reporting with regard to Hudson's illness is perhaps illustrated most clearly in some of the headlines found in the popular newspapers, e.g. 'Rock Hudson – living the Hollywood lie', which made oblique reference to the misleading nature of his strongly heterosexual image. It needs to be said that the 'quality' newspapers were not entirely free of sensation-seeking headlines and in at least one, made even more personal reference to Hudson's private life, e.g. 'Hollywood gays rally to Hudson' (*Guardian* 27 July 1985).

As discussed below, even if the press rarely has the power to influence behaviour directly, it can nevertheless serve to raise the public consciousness on certain issues through its agenda-setting activities (McCombs and Shaw, 1972). With regard to AIDS, much of the early press coverage encouraged victim-blaming through its concentration on homosexuals (Naylor, 1985) and intravenous drug users as the main contenders for contracting the disease. This could hardly be said to have prepared the way for the later government pronouncements that any sexually active individual is potentially at risk. Indeed, it may at least partially explain why, in spite of the barrage of government-backed campaigning, certain sectors of the population – in particular, it would seem, young, sexual active men – are taking no heed of these warnings (*SCAN*, April 1987).

The evidence presented in the previous sections supports the proposal made by Kristiansen and Harding (1988) that the lower socioeconomic groups in society not only receive less health information, but the health information they are presented with is less 'useful'. By 'useful' is meant that the information is of an educational nature and comes from reputable sources. Furthermore, the issues which directly concern the more deprived groups in society are not being discussed in their newspapers. Kristiansen and Harding cite this inequality in health information as another example of the inequalities in health that exist in Britain. Indeed, they suggest that the press may be a contributory factor to the inequalities in distribution of morbidity and premature mortality across social classes.

Regional Differences in Press Coverage of Health Issues

In a comparative study of the UK national, Scottish national and Scottish local press, there was found to be considerable variation in the coverage given to health issues (Currie, 1987). Table 4.5 shows the mean number of health articles per paper in each group of newspapers during July 1985. The table indicates that readers of a Scottish national newspaper receive less health information than readers of a UK national paper and, furthermore, that those individuals who read only a Scottish local paper are even less adequately served.

Table 4.5
Mean Number of Health-Related Articles per Type of
Newspaper, July 1985

UK national	Scottish national	Scottish local
(n=3)	(n=5)	(n=4)
124	101	80

Scotland is renowned for its poor record on morbidity and mortality from the major chronic diseases of coronary heart disease and lung cancer, and for its high smoking rates and alcohol-related problems (General Register Office, 1987). Intuitively, it might be expected that there would be a correspondingly high profile given to health issues in the Scottish press. Instead, there would appear to be a notable absence of health from the agenda. Once again, inequalities in health information would appear to be correlated with, and may even contribute to, inequalities in health, in this case inequalities being on a regional or north south basis.

The role of community development in changing the public health is discussed in Chapter 8. The idea is that action for change is located at the level of the community rather than nationally and that it is controlled by the members of the community themselves. Local newspapers could potentially play a key role in publicizing initiatives of this kind. As shown in an earlier section, the press and television tend to use and re-use the doctor-hospital-technology framework for discussing health issues. In local papers there is a need to discard such images and to frame issues within the context of the community and its particular health problems.

The Process of Communication: Capturing the Audience's Attention

A number of different measures have been used to assess the interest that the press takes in particular issues; the most commonly employed is the number of column inches for example Best *et al.* (1977) used column inches to measure press coverage of the newly published DHSS document entitled *Prevention and Health: Everybody's Business* (DHSS, 1976) and compare it to the coverage given to other issues. Column inches were also used to compare coverage of the 1983 'pill scare' in the national and provincial newspapers (Wellings, 1985).

Column inches is a rather crude measure with which to compare coverage of an issue by different newspapers since newspapers vary in page size and, from day to day, in their number of pages. To overcome this problem Kristiansen and Harding (1988) calculated the relative amount of total newspaper space devoted to particular health issues when comparing health coverage in the large-format quality press with that in the popular tabloids.

Headlines are used by the reader to scan and select which articles he will read, and it has been shown experimentally that the larger the headline, the more likely that it, and the article that follows, will be read (Knapper and Warr, 1965). The popular press typically use larger headlines than the quality press (McQuail, 1976). This is illustrated in Welling's (1985) paper on the press coverage of the *Lancet's* articles by Vessey *et al.*

(1983) and Pike *et al.* (1983) linking the oral contraceptive pill to cervical and breast cancer respectively. The headlines which appeared in the popular press such as the *Sun* and the *Standard* were considerably taller and bolder than those in quality papers such as *The Times* and *The Guardian.*

Headlines not only attract attention, but their wording may influence the interpretation of the story that follows. Tannenbaum (1953) showed this to be the case in a laboratory experiment, but under conditions that can hardly be said to have mimicked closely the typical daily newspaper reading situation. Nevertheless, if a headline is particularly sensational it is possible that its message might affect the meaning taken from the rest of the article in a 'real-life' situation. Headlines such as 'Women on the pill face new cancer fear' *(Daily Star* 21 October 1983) could easily lead to hurried and uncritical scanning of the article, especially where already existing fears are apparently being confirmed in print. Unfortunately, it is rather difficult to test such a hypothesis except under somewhat unrealistic conditions, and then the problem remains of how far one can extrapolate from the findings to reality.

Position on the page and location in the newspaper are also thought to be important in determining the likelihood of an article being read. Budd (1964) interviewed newspaper editors to ascertain which criteria were most important in giving an article prominence. The editors agreed that that placement above the fold (i.e. in the top half of the page, gave an article more newsplay, as did the article's location on the front page, an editorial page or another 'departmental' page. Budd's survey was somewhat limited, with only eight editors being interviewed; furthermore, there was no scientific basis for their opinions – they were simply founded in observation and experience. Having said this, laboratory experiments conducted to investigate the importance of article position to the readership (Knapper and Warr, 1965b) gave rather inconclusive results which illustrate the difficulty of simulating a day-to-day activity such as newspaper-reading in the laboratory.

Programme length and time of broadcasting are probably the best indicators of the prominence that television producers wish to give to a particular issue. However, there are constraints which will influence the coverage that can be given, and these constraints will differ according to the type of programme. As discussed previously television coverage takes several forms: news, documentary, magazine/educational and drama. In the news, those items considered by the production team to be the most important and dramatic (and not necessarily in that order) appear early on in the programme. As far as health is concerned the dramatic stories tend to cover issues such as a breakthrough in the development of a new drug, surgical procedure or other medical treatment; an outbreak of disease such as legionnaires' or salmonella or the illness of a famous person, for example, Ronald Reagan's colorectal cancer in 1985. Prevention generally does not hit the headlines unless the disease concerned can be sensationalized in some way; AIDS is an example where considerable newsplay has been made from the fact that it is sexual behaviour and drug-taking behaviour that must be altered if contracting the disease is to be avoided.

Documentaries and other educational programmes tend to be produced in series broadcast at a viewing time chosen so as to cater for the potential audience. Viewer's attention will be drawn to the programme by prior publicity.

In soap opera, and other drama, some producers do seem to recognize that they have a role to play in providing useful health information but expect the audience to use their own judgement and do not see themselves as having any responsibility since they are dealing in entertainment not education and put the plot before the accurate portrayal of reality (Daintree, 1986).

Factors Affecting Health Coverage by the Media: Conclusions

There are forces operating that determine which health issues become news and which are overlooked by the media. In the selection process, health-related issues not only compete for attention with non-health issues, but there is also competition within the total pool of potentially reportable health issues. This double selection process has been examined in relation to crime news (Roshier, 1976) and it is thought that it is important in shaping the 'official' picture of crime. Images of health portrayed by the media are similarly shaped by the processes of selection and omission.

In his analysis of the selection for publication of crime news Roshier found that certain characteristics were favoured for example, the involvement of a famous person, sentimental/dramatic circumstances. The research findings on media health coverage described in earlier sections suggest that the same may be true for health news as in the high profile given in the British press to drug abuse, and to AIDS when contracted by a famous film star, and the rather low profile given to social factors in ill health and to prevention in the press and in television medical programmes.

The operational constraints on news production mean that it is easier to describe events that occur within the period of a day, or can be made to sound as if they do. Health issues of a more complex and long-standing nature would, therefore, tend to be rejected in favour of an exciting event. So, for example, an article on social deprivation and its effects on health may be not be published where the story of a young transplant patient would be.

In addition to the operational constraints there are the ideational constraints which are more difficult to pin down since they are to a large extent hidden. They would perhaps be more easily characterized by those articles that never get written or, if written, never get published; however, these constraints have to be inferred from any bias that can be seen in what does emerge on the printed page or on the television screen. Murdoch (1974) proposed that the meaning system adhered to by the media reflects that of the dominant groups in society and is illustrated by the fact that journalists tend to use images and interpretive frameworks which are consonant with that meaning system. It has been suggested by Farrant and Russell (1986) that as far as health education/promotion is concerned the 'official position', or accepted conceptual framework, is one which advocates health education for individual change and tends to neglect the issues of deprivation and inequalities in health. They contend that the health messages avoid any suggestion of social action and oversimplify complex and difficult issues.

Media Effects

Before discussing the role of the mass media in influencing the public health through raising awareness or more directly affecting attitudes, beliefs or behaviour, the various models that have been developed to explain media effects are examined. The earlier studies of the mass media were based on the idea that their effects were simple and direct (Glover, 1984), for example, violence on television would incite violence in viewers. This 'hypodermic syringe' model was rejected when it became clear that audiences are not simply passive recipients of the media's messages and indeed, are selective and make judgements as to the validity of what they read, see and hear. The two-step flow model, the dominant paradigm until the late 1970s was also ultimately rejected for its oversimplistic notion that audiences could be divided into active and passive members; the active members or opinion leaders were supposed to be influenced by the media and in turn influence the passive members of society (Glover, 1984).

In the third model to be proposed, the 'uses and gratifications' model, the members of the audience were at last recognized as having a more important role. They were seen as using the media to satisfy individual needs and interests. The model, however, lacked any broader societal perspective; a criticism that cannot be levelled at the final model discussed here, the 'cultural effects' model (Glover, 1984). This model portrays the media as having a key role in creating a set of beliefs and values which the members of the audience use to help them to understand the society in which they live. The main difference between this model and the earlier ones is that it takes into account that the images used by the media will be interpreted according to the particular social circumstances and belief system of the audience. The model attempts to bring together both the way in which meanings are created by the media and the way in which these relate differently to the cultures of the particular groups [Glover, 1984).

Media effects on the public health may be visualized as a continuum from subtle influences on people's understanding and knowledge concerning particular health issues, to more direct influences on health-related behaviour. Media effects are notoriously difficult to study because of the problems of teasing out media effects from other influences which arise in the context of a network of family, work and other social contacts.

Efforts have been made to determine the media's role and two main types of methodologies have been employed in researching media effects. One approach may be described as epidemiological: following a particular event which is reported on the front page of the newspapers or in a special television documentary, indicators of a change in the health behaviour of the population are sought and measured. Examples of indicators include the fall in prescriptions for oral contraceptives after the 'pill scare' in 1983 (Wellings, 1985), and the decrease in kidneys donated after a BBC documentary questioning the criteria used to determine brain death (Bradley and Brooman, 1980). Obviously, this is a somewhat opportunistic approach. A more satisfactory way of studying responses to media output could be through continuous monitoring of health-related behaviour and behavioural change in the population, so that the impact of significant media events would be recorded. The Research Unit in Health and Behavioural Change of the University of Edinburgh (RUHBC) is currently developing a computerized system that will facilitate the collection of longitudinal data on the population. If media events are recorded at the same time then it should be possible to link changes in knowledge, attitudes and behaviour to media coverage of health issues.

The other main approach used to study media effects is experimental in design. This methodology has been employed to examine, for example, the effects of headline size and page layout on subjects' reading and understanding of newspaper articles (see above). Morley (1980) also used an experimental approach to investigate variation in audience response to television broadcasts. He showed video recordings of a daily magazine programme, 'Nationwide', to 29 different sets of subjects. Afterwards, discussions were held in the groups in order to examine their responses. This type of research is useful for revealing immediate responses to media output and in Morley's study showed that audiences are not uniform in their responses. However, it is obviously not suitable for investigating longer-term effects on attitudes or behaviour.

There are examples, mentioned above, which suggest that the media may have direct effects on behaviour. At first glance they seem to lend support to the 'hypodermic syringe' model described in the previous section. Using the example of the 'pill scare' it can be shown that this would be a somewhat superficial interpretation of events. Following press coverage, described earlier, of two papers that appeared in the *Lancet* suggesting that the oral contraceptive pill was a risk factor for breast cancer and cervical cancer, there was a significant decrease in pill use as indicated by the reduction in prescriptions being written in England and Wales (Wellings, 1985). The findings, however, could also be interpreted within the framework of the cultural effects model. Not all women who read the press coverage stopped taking the pill. This could be interpreted as evidence that, depending on the particular experiential and educational characteristics of the women, their response to reading the media output would be different. Of course, this is speculative, but points to the kinds of questions that should be asked when studies of media effects are being conducted.

There are relatively few examples of direct media effects on the health behaviour of audiences. Most health-related behavioural change is a slow complex process as described in the next chapter. The role of the media, therefore, may be one of creating a climate supportive to change, for example, by providing useful information and by creating positive images relating to improvements in health resulting from change. However, in reality, the media often present contradictory images which are not supportive to health-enhancing behaviour. One of the main ways in which they do this is through their alliance with commercial interests: by advertising cigarettes they contradict any media coverage they have given to the adverse health effects of smoking. By the use of persuasive imagery young women have been successfully targeted by the tobacco companies; in spite of the fact that women's magazines often deplore smoking in their health columns, some of them still provide space for cigarette advertisements on the adjacent pages (Amos, 1984).

The information content of media health coverage is obviously crucial in relation to its usefulness to individuals who are interested in improving their health or reducing their chances of ill health. Often the media oversimplify issues which are complex and controversial. For example, whilst the media have focused on individual eating habits in the link between diet and heart disease, they have tended to ignore the epidemiological evidence of regional differences in heart disease which suggests that it has a more complex aetiology and is unlikely to be prevented at an individual level through a simple change of diet (Farrant and Russell, 1986). Breast cancer screening is another issue where the surrounding controversy may be ignored by the media. Breast screening itself does not prevent breast cancer, and indeed its general usefulness is in debate (Skrabanek, 1985). Yet its portrayal by the media may very often be couched in such terms as to suggest that it is of unquestionable benefit to women. Superficial treatment by the media of complex issues may be counterproductive in the long term. Public scepticism may result and rebound adversely on the outcome of future campaigns in which important health information is being presented, such as the AIDS campaign.

Most media influences are likely to be subtle and therefore difficult to study. Raising of the public's consciousness is usually inferred but rarely demonstrated to be a result of the agenda-setting activities of the media. Surveys can ask the public where they gained their information about particular health-related issues. Few will deny that 'they heard something about it on TV.' This scarcely provides hard evidence for the media's role in health promotion. Perhaps researchers will have to be content with the notion that the media clearly constitute a force in shaping health beliefs but that cultural, experiential and social environmental factors have an equal if not more influential role in changing the public health.

CHAPTER 5

Health-Related Behavioural Change

In recent years official strategies for changing the public health have focused almost exclusively on the behaviour or 'life styles' of individuals. As subsequent chapters will suggest, there are empirical reasons why these strategies are misguided in their assumption that the interacting complex of aetiological factors can be reduced to so simple a formula. This chapter will describe the premises upon which attempts to change the behaviour of the public are based and examine the theoretical and methodological reasons for their largely ineffectual impact. It will then go on to outline the principles of a new theory of behaviour change.

The assumptions underlying the majority of health education and health promotion strategies, whether presented via the mass media, in face-to-face situations or in community campaigns, are threefold:

—that human beings are primarily rational beings;
—that provided with sensible information about the desirability of change they will follow it; and .
—that behavioural change can be brought about without consideration of the context in which the behaviour occurs.

Neither experience, history nor experiment supports these premises.

Attempts to change health-related behaviours by health educators and others have largely failed due to their undue reliance on the literature of social psychology and the application of models of behavioural change which owe more to the cooperation of American college students than they do to an understanding of the context and complexity of the phenomenon itself.

Although humans are capable of rational thought and even of apparently rational behaviour, it is doubtful if this is a preferred mode of operating for more than a minority or for more than limited periods of time. Moreover, thought is not necessarily a precursor of behaviour. Rather, action is a consequence not solely of cognition but also of that mix of emotion, habit, impulse, bloody-mindedness and lack of forethought which is characteristically human.

The development of behaviour forms a major part of human adaptation involving cognitive organization, perception, the construction of meaning and the creation of a coherent personal world. In addition, neurological and physiological changes are involved at the level of learning, monitoring and pattern recognition.

It is thus evident that the daily activities of an individual form an integral part of that individual's physiological, social and psychological being. Patterns of behaviour of an apparently discrete kind – e.g. eating, are, in fact, integrated into a constant flow of amalgamated activities. Change in such patterns is both a consequence and a cause of other fluctuations in activity.

Models for changing behaviour are obviously of great interest to all those who have a professional stake in bringing about a particular state of affairs, whether this be political, social, economic or medical, but the academic discipline which has dominated the field of behavioural change is psychology, and some of the problematic aspects of attempts to develop change strategies for health relate to the fact that since the 1920s academic psychology has adopted a positivist philosophy. Human beings have been viewed as objects much like any other object, animate or inanimate, of scientific experimentation. This has led to the unfortunate consequence of selected bits of behaviour being treated as isolated and discrete actions, such that given a set of dependent variables certain events are assumed to follow regardless of context.

Several formulae for behavioural change have been drawn up over the years, some of which have been utilized by health educators and, now, health promotion promoters, in attempts to influence health-related behaviour. Although these models differ somewhat in their terms and perspectives they have in common fundamental methodological and theoretical shortcomings and pay little attention to economic, political and structural constraints on behaviour or indeed to the realities of everyday life. Nor do they give much credit to individual interpretation, innovation or circumstances.

Models of Behavioural Change

There are basically three types of studies within psychology which have behavioural change as their objective and which have been used to structure strategies for changing health-related behaviour. These are the social influence model, attitudinal models and behaviourism.

Studies of social influence have been dominated by the concept of conformity, that is, the notion that a great deal of individual behaviour tends towards the normative. Thus, faced with a discrepancy between his or her own actions and those of a relevant group, the individual will tend to change in the direction of the group norm. Conformity has been subdivided into compliance, that is, public acceptance but private autonomy; identification, that is, temporary acceptance of group mores during a period of close contact with a particular group; and internalization, that is, private and public conformity to group values (Kelman, 1969). The degree to which behaviour changes in the face of group pressure is said to be related to demographic variables, the strength of the original behaviour, the number of supporters and personality factors (Kiesler and Kiesler, 1969). Conformity has been explained in terms of a social comparison process which maintains the flimsy fabric of social reality. Since there is no true yardstick for most beliefs and behaviours, no 'right' or 'wrong', except as they manifest themselves in contemporary usage, a person who is unsure of the correct way to behave will do as he or she thinks those around are doing. Of course, it is evident that normative patterns do develop which govern to some extent acceptable and non-acceptable behaviour One of the triumphs of anti-smoking campaigns has been to make cigarette smoking into a largely 'deviant' behaviour in contrast to the situation 30 years ago. However, although the concept of conformity is easily applied to general phenomena it is hard to detect it at an individual level since any behaviour is not an isolated set of actions susceptible to clearly defined situations, but rather part of an integrated social dynamic. Similar criticisms can be made of other concepts such as 'obedience to authority' (Milgram, 1974) and 'deindividuation' (Zimbardo, 1970), where behavioural change can be demonstrated under highly artificial conditions, but where explanatory variables cannot be extrapolated into everyday life.

Other studies of social influence have concentrated on 'modelling' effects. These refer to a tendency to imitate other people, particularly under conditions of uncertainty. Bandura (1969) has proposed three types of modelling effects: inhibitory or disinhibitory, when the actions of others strengthen or weaken the restraints of an observer against performing a particular act; response-facilitating effects, which enhance tendencies already present; and observational learning effects, where a person may acquire a potential behaviour merely by observation and without immediate imitation. The principles of social modelling underlie the use of rock stars, footballers and other celebrities in health education campaigns. Again, however, the sequelae of exposure to models are highly unpredictable except under the isolated and static laboratory-type conditions of the psychological experiment.

Studies of social influence as a trigger to behavioural change have been based largely on *in vitro* experiments which have used college students as subjects. Most of the work, moreover, has its origins in the United States, where students are obliged to participate in experiments or where volunteers have been paid. These conditions alone are sufficient to call into question the validity of the results of most of the studies, whatever the spurious appeal of the situations from which they arise.

The work of Kurt Lewin, however, particularly in relation to group influences, has been set in a wider context of social processes and social management. Lewin's studies were founded in *Gestalt* theory which treats behaviour, not as a 'thing', but as a process. Attempts to influence the food habits of housewives during World War II showed that active participation in the group process and a public commitment to change were more effective in the long term than was a situation where individuals were passively subjected to information (Lewin, 1947). Lewin discussed the kinds and direction of the forces required to 'unfreeze' social habits from a state of 'quasi-stationary equilibrium' and ways in which new behaviours could be prevented from relapsing by re-freezing' them into permanency. These requirements he saw as being met primarily by the forces present in group dynamics. The work of Lewin and his colleagues represents one of the relatively rare attempts to derive research from a clearly stated theoretical stance.

The word 'attitude' is highly ambiguous. It means nothing and everything. It is a word in general parlance as well as having a variety of definitions in psychological and sociological literature The concept of attitude has played an important role in social psychology for decades, possibly for its usefulness as a portmanteau containing shreds of ideas and layers of prejudice which are rarely, if ever, unpacked. Attitudes have been variously defined as beliefs, dispositions, tendencies, evaluations, likes and dislikes, but, more relevantly for the purposes of this chapter also as compositions of affective, cognitive and behavioural elements (Wagner, 1969).

This amalgam of behaviour, knowledge and feelings under the rubric of the term 'attitude' has generated a great deal of useless research and irrelevant activity in many areas, including health education, because it has led to the misconceived idea that changing knowledge and/or feelings will somehow change behaviour. Reviews by Gatherer *et al.* (1979) and Wenzel (1983) attest to the ineffectual nature of this notion.

The voluminous literature on this topic reports a great many studies of 'attitudes' and behaviour and demonstrates that the relationship between the concepts of attitude as a hypothetical construct and as observable action is uncertain. Practical attempts, both to measure the attitudes of the general public and to try to change their attitudes by means of persuasive communications have been based upon two assumptions:

—that there is something known as an attitude which can be measured in the same way as one can measure, say, a piece of land; and
—that there exist certain combinations of key words and actions which will trigger off a change in attitude among members of the public.

Attitudes are virtually always inferred from verbal statements, written or spoken, collected by questionnaires, interviews, scaling methods, or any combination of these, many of which are of doubtful, often untested, reliability and validity. This approach, in turn, raises a number of methodological problems:

1. *The definition of just what it is that is meant by an attitude.*   Most social psychologists see attitude as a global term for a coalescence of behaviour, emotion and cognition. Attempts have been made to measure all three, say in relation to smoking habits (Marsh, 1985; Uutela, 1986). However, the idea that the components are separate means that once they are externalized from the individuals concerned there is no way in which they can be recombined to give an accurate reflection of the position of any individual on that particular issue.
2. *The nature of the relationship between overt verbal response and behaviour*   Most studies have shown that what people say is not necessarily a guide to what they will do, probably because opinion and action are influenced by a different set of antecedent and situational variables (Kuter *et al.*, 1952; Wrightsman, 1966; La Pierre, 1934; Wicker, 1971).
3. *The relationship between a score on a questionnaire or scale and the respondent's tendency to act*   This relationship is probably even more remote than that between opinion and behaviour.

As with studies of social influence, attempts to change attitudes have been based upon highly artificial situations rather than upon evidence from 'naturally occurring' events. Biases of education, class, culture and willingness to participate are built into most attitude research. Hypothetical concepts such as 'cognitive dissonance (Festinger, 1957) are used to 'explain' why certain types of result are obtained, leading to the unfortunate result that 'cognitive dissonance' has sometimes been reified as something which 'really exists' in the mind of a person, instead of being merely a *post hoc* justification (Brown, 1965).

Fishbein and Ajzen (1975) have focused upon beliefs rather than attitudes as basic determinants of behaviour, arguing that if beliefs about the consequences of certain behaviours can be changed this will lead to a change in evaluation of the behaviours. In addition, it is said that influencing beliefs about the individual's expectations of specific referents will affect subjective norms. Thus, theoretically, behavioural change should follow from influencing salient beliefs in a population and introducing new beliefs. These authors introduce the concept of 'intention' and the degree to which intentions to perform actions are under attitudinal or normative control. Although this model receives some support in that beliefs and intentions are sometimes predictive of behaviour, it cannot account for the fact that often they are not. Again, the failure to take the context of behaviour into account is a major drawback.

The effects of various aspects of persuasive communications on attitudes have also received a good deal of attention, e.g. the credibility of the source, one-sided versus two-sided messages, the order of presenting information, arousal of emotions, especially fear arousal, and the characteristics of the audience (Hovland *et al.*, 1949; Elms, 1972; Leventhal *et al.*, 1967; Janis and Field, 1956). The results of research have been inconclusive and, in general, suggest that whilst subjects exposed to a persuasive communication may sometimes change their expressed opinions, the effects on behaviour are largely unpredictable both in direction and duration.

The behavioural model actually contains a number of disparate theoretical approaches, including classical conditioning, operant conditioning and cognitive behaviour modification. From humble but singular beginnings associated with cats releasing themselves from boxes, pigeons learning to play table tennis and rats running in mazes, behaviour modification is now one of the most used forms of attempts to control and change behaviour, particularly in strategies of treatment for health problems (King and Remenyi, 1986).

Put at its simplest, the behavioural model has as its premise that behaviour develops through contingencies of reward and punishment. Certain acts are reinforced because they, or their consequences, are associated with a rewarding experience, which may be physical pleasure or psychological benefits such as enhanced self-esteem. Some rewards may be the mere absence of adverse consequences. Obversely, actions which are 'punished' either directly or by the withholding of some reward will tend to die out. Such techniques are used, for example, in desensitizing people to phobias, alleviating chronic pain, treating enuresis and discouraging smoking, with varying degrees of success (Horne and McCormack, 1984; Peck, 1982; Ciminero and Doleys, 1976; Lichtenstein, 1982). The architect of behaviourism, B. F. Skinner, seemed to believe that most of the ills of society could be removed by a judicious control of reinforcement strategies (Skinner, 1948).

The behavioural approach focuses on current rather than historical determinants of behaviour, and ignores the wider social context of the behaviour. It thus aims to treat a specific set of actions in isolation by manipulation of environmental contingencies, as in aversion therapy and desensitization techniques.

Health-Related Behavioural Change

The foregoing models, alone or in a variety of combinations, have been used in attempts by health education and health promotion agencies to change behaviour supposedly related to health status: primarily, smoking, alcohol and illicit drug use, diet and exercise. The underlying rationale for this is that certain patterns of these behaviours constitute risk factors for a variety of diseases, in particular, lung cancer and cardiovascular disease. (The fact that the distribution of such diseases, controlling for the behaviours in question, is not equally spread throughout the population, but, rather, tends to concentrate geographically and by social class, will be addressed later.) Consequently, strategies have been developed which purport to persuade the public to change their behaviour. These strategies have been applied in four areas: (a) at individual or 'treatment level, (b) at group level, (c) at community level, (d) in the mass media.

Individual level

These attempts at influencing behaviour may be regarded as forms of 'treatment' since they generally involve the participation of volunteers in some quasi-therapeutic regime, with close supervision, under intensive regimens based upon the principles of behaviourism. Such regimens have generally been applied to alcohol abusers, smokers and the overweight.

In general, although most such programmes show limited short-term change, the evidence for long-term change is scant and their effectiveness in many cases seems comparable to that of no treatment at all. For example, it has been noted, in relation to treatment for alcohol problems, that not one of the dozens of formal treatments for alcoholism appears to be either necessary or sufficient for recovery (Emrick, 1980). Similarly, for narcotic addiction, Callahan (1980) concluded that all known forms of intervention were relatively ineffective. Attempts to find successful cessation methods for cigarette-smokers have also largely failed (McFall, 1978). In a national sample of the population of the United States it was found that about half the number of current smokers had considered stopping, a third had tried to stop, 15% had achieved short-term success and 7.5% had stopped for months or over; a state of affairs which would seem to indicate a high level of motivation combined with a low measure of success (Horn, 1968). (This study also casts doubt on the reliability of figures pertaining to the number of people who have stopped smoking. 'Snapshot' studies are likely to seriously overestimate the numbers because of transitory attempts to quit.)

Treatments involving psychological principles seem to follow a similar pattern of sound rationale and conscientious activity, but conclude with modest levels of success as indicated in reviews of obesity (Leon, 1976; Ley, 1977), smoking (Raw, 1977; Leventhal and Geary', 1980), alcohol (Emrick, 1980; Oxford and Edwards, 1977) and drug use (Kurland, 1978). In most cases where follow-up has taken place, the success rate is around one-third at 6 to 12 months and further relapse is probably to be expected. This level appears to be largely independent of the particular treatment applied.

A more complex approach to risk factors utilizes Health Hazard Risk Appraisal and contains a five-age process of progress towards behavioural change:

1 An individual is made aware of a risk to his or her own health because of some behaviour. or behaviours and/or personal characteristics.
2 The individual accepts at-risk status.
3 This knowledge is integrated into self-images.
4 Efforts to change are made.
5 The individual applies knowledge to the process of change (Brown, 1976).

In general, the results of this approach are equivocal: it does, however, seem to provide a stimulus to change for some people, especially in relation to exercise, weight control and reduced alcohol intake (Milsum *et al.*, 1976; Warner, 1977; Lauzon, 1977).

Those regimens of individual treatment which have been reasonably successful provide useful pointers to the necessary elements for behavioural change. For example, individuals have to stay with the programme and struggle with change. Efforts are most likely to be successful where skills learned in the programme are transferable to the everyday context and where the individual is supported by family members and signifi-cant others (Witschi *et al.*, 1978; Brownell *et al.*, 1979; Mahoney and Mahoney, 1976). Successful change needs to be followed by a 'maintenance' period during which the new behaviour is reinforced (Benfari *et al.*, 1981). Role-playing involving emotional outburst has proved efficacious (Janis and Mann, 1965) and rehearsal, both imagined and real, of the new behaviour seems to help (Cohen *et al.*, 1979). Self-management procedures where the clients assume major responsibility for changes, set their own personal objectives, monitor their own behaviour and evaluate their own success, are more likely to result in the completion of a regimen (McFall, 1970; Champlin and Karoly, 1975).

Group influence

Group techniques have been used to apparently good effect with weight watchers and in Alcoholics Anonymous. Both situations involve a certain amount of initial confession, identification with the values and aims of the group, peer reinforcement, public commit-ment and social support. However, the success of weight watchers' groups appears to be very limited in the long term (Leon, 1976) and it is impossible to estimate the success of Alcoholics Anonymous since research studies are discouraged. The drop-out rate is known to be high. Rather more reliable information is available from health education attempts at the worksite.

Several studies have suggested a limited measure of success for workplace health education and promotion. For example, the STAYWELL programme in the USA focuses on long-term changes in health behaviour, particularly smoking, weight control, diet and stress management. Employees are given orientation to the programme, assess-ment of their health-related behaviours, health hazard appraisal and the opportunity to participate in various courses. In addition, volunteers engage in discussing and then modifying aspects of the work environment and normative behaviours which are related to health, e.g. availability of nutritious food, initiating sporting activities. Support groups in which employees help each other change target behaviours are formed (Naditch, 1984). Evaluation of the effectiveness of this programme indicates that a certain amount of change is produced, particularly in smoking, weight control and exercise. Other similar programmes also suggest a limited amount of change (Nathan, 1984; Carrington *et al.*, 1980; Fitness Systems Inc., 1980). Blair *et al.* (1984) reported that an evaluation of behavioural change in teachers who participated in a 10-week health promotion programme carried out in the school, which emphasized exercise, stress management and nutrition showed that they were more likely to increase levels of vigorous exercise, lose weight, lower blood pressure and report a higher level of well-being than compar-able control groups. A notable feature of these programmes is that they take place within a context which is familiar and meaningful to the participants and, unlike many other attempts at influence involve the targets of the programme in influencing others like themselves.

Some of the evaluations of group and worksite interventions must be suspect, subject as they are to volunteer bias and demand characteristics. However, there is little doubt that some changes in behaviour are produced, particularly when active participation is demanded, the context is a familiar one, normative processes are engaged and social support is available.

Community campaigns

Adoption of a community setting for planned intervention is becoming increasingly popular. One of the best known community-based programmes is the North Karelia project which aimed at changing behaviours related to the risk of cardiovascular disease, in conjunction with changes in health services delivery and modifications in the environment, such as smoking restrictions, and encouraging the sale of low-fat products. Strategies for change involved local authorities and community groups in the promotion of, for example, no-smoking areas, the dissemination of information and the establishment of networks of lay leaders trained to support activities in the community. Surveys showed that health behaviours and associated risk factors changed in the desired direction over a 10-year period (Puska et al., 1981, 1983; Vartiainen et al., 1986.) However, similar changes took place outside the target area which suggested difficulties in disaggregating the effects of the specific programme from larger effects in the country as a whole, including a general improvement in social conditions in Finland. Other similar projects are under way in the United States, e.g. the Minnesota Heart Health Program (Blackburn et al., 1984) and the Pawtucket experiment (Abrams et al., 1981). Evaluative data from the latter indicate changes in response to screening attendance after a 2-month period (Lefebvre et al., 1986).

One of the most interesting programmes of this type was the Multiple Risk Factor Intervention Trial (MRFIT), which involved a randomized design, where the experimental group was subjected to special intervention including group discussion, counseling, involvement of family members and a commitment to change on the part of the participants. After 7 years, 40% of smokers had stopped and 64% of hypertensives had successfully controlled their blood pressure. Unfortunately for the credibility of the interventions similar results were also observed in the control group, many of whom also changed their behaviour without the benefit of the interventions. The resources applied in the MRFIT trial represent, the best available strategies for maximizing behavioural change, but as such, must be regarded as still decidedly deficient (MRFIT Research Group, 1982).

This kind of project is clearly very expensive, both financially and in terms of personnel. In addition, whatever the strategy employed, the model is still one of imposing need for change from outside the community, and then persuading people that change is, indeed, desirable.

A different approach is taken by community development initiatives, such as the one described in Chapter 8. Based upon the Declaration of Alma-Ata, that the public should be encouraged to articulate their own health-related needs and provided with the opportunity of critically examining and meeting those needs in ways they consider appropriate, this approach acknowledges that attempts to change individual behaviour in relation to, say, smoking, alcohol or food habits are often of little interest to people struggling to get by on low incomes in the face of many day-to-day problems.

The objectives of most community health projects in the UK are two-fold: encouraging active involvement by the community in health care, and encouraging the local health service to be more responsive to health needs. Evaluation of such projects in terms of behavioural change is very difficult, for the effects appear to be diffuse and often outside traditional outcome measures. However, there is evidence that behavioural changes occur, often as a result of participation in local self-help groups and as a consequence of active involvement in organizing campaigns, courses and management groups. The operation of a Well Woman Clinic in Manchester, for example led to very high levels of utilization especially by working-class women and those over 43 years of age, groups normally underrepresented in their use of preventive services. Important factors in the success of the clinic were the equal participation of lay people and medical staff, collective decision-making, an informal atmosphere and the giving of equal weight to traditionally 'non-medical' issues such as housing and poor self-esteem (CPF, 1983).

Mass media campaigns

These have been alluded to in the previous chapter. Suffice it to say that the ostensible purpose of mass media campaigns in health education is to educate the public about risks and benefits of various health-related behaviours. More often, however, such campaigns present an over-simplified version of the information available and thus have more the appearance of propaganda. Such campaigns are mostly aimed at the general public via television and/or radio and the press. Occasionally specific groups are targeted – pregnant women, young people, the overweight. Techniques include the use of role models, emotive messages and appeals to conformist tendencies.

Evaluations of such campaigns usually show a short term increase in knowledge for a minority of the audience. Success in changing behaviour is most apparent, albeit meagre, where a single clear action is recommended but there is little evidence of long-term change except where campaigns are continued for periods of over 12 months, when about 10 per cent of the targeted population can be expected to show changes in behaviour (Gatherer et al., 1979).

The most likely effect of media campaigns is that they play a part in the slow change which takes place over a period of years by altering the climate of opinion, thus making people more susceptible to other influences. An evaluation of the effects of the 'So you want to stop smoking?' series broadcast on British television suggested that the series had some success in influencing the intention of smokers to stop smoking, although this was not, at the time, predictive of actual behaviour (Hallett and Sutton, 1986).

It has been pointed out that, in the USA, health education, like medical technology, demonstrates high cost for low returns. Millions of dollars have been spent on trying to persuade people to change their habits in relation to smoking, diet, drugs and alcohol, exercise and driving, without notable success, although some changes have occurred in a minority of the population (Cohen and Cohen, 1978). Although a smaller proportion of the health budget is spent on health education in Britain, the outcome appears to be much the same.

It should be noted that very few evaluative studies of attempts to change health-related behaviour meet the essential criteria for relating independent and dependent variables. These are that alterations in behaviour, rather than knowledge attitudes or intention, should be the outcome indicators and that rigorous research designs with control groups, or at least good comparison groups, should be used. The few studies that have demonstrated these criteria show that traditional health education strategies have no more than a minimum effect on behaviour (Haggerty, 1977). Moreover, the lack of firm theoretical guidelines prohibits aggregation and means that cumulative data are not available, so that strategies accumulate piecemeal without systematic testing.

It should be noted that many of the models upon which health education strategies are built implicitly adopt a mechanistic orientation, whereby individuals are seen as responding to forces in the environment which push them or pull on them. Human behaviour, however, may equally well be explained by reference to the person as self directed and self-monitoring, acting with awareness within complex, meaningful interactions with other people and the environment, as has been argued in Chapter 3.

Self-Initiated Change

Overall, it can be said that research evidence shows a distinct lack of significant success in linking behavioural changes to planned interventions, and yet it is demonstrably true that behaviours in a population do change quite markedly over time.

A report by the Royal College of Physicians (1977) documented the dramatic change in the smoking habits of some groups, and Horn (1972) estimated that about 13 million smokers quit between 1966 and 1970 and that 99 % did so without any form of official help. A long-term follow-up of problem drinkers found that two-thirds had modified their drinking without outside intervention (Valliant, 1983).

The recognition that health-related activities are intimately bound to existential and structural systems has been belatedly acknowledged in the new term 'health promotion'. Indeed, the recent promotion of 'health promotion' seems to be based, at least in part, on a tacit acknowledgement of the failure of conventional health education to demonstrate any significant direct links between its various activities and campaigns and changes in health-related behaviour (Wenzel, 1983; Gathereret et al., 1977). It seems that an understanding of how behaviour changes in the context of everyday activities and adaptations would provide a more enlightening and practical basis for planned interventions. There has been remarkably little work carried out on 'self-initiated' behavioural change and few attempts to study such change systematically. Where such studies have been done they highlight some important issues, such as the role of precipitating life-events, the minor part played by health concerns and the major contribution of social context.

Studies of modification or cessation of alcohol use have found that change is usually preceded by some personal crisis which brings the drinking into sharp focus. Tuchfeld (1981) documents instances of a sudden change in drinking habits which is activated by social phenomena. For example, a pregnant woman gave up alcohol when she felt her baby quiver as she took a drink; a man stopped drinking when his father died because he attributed the death to alcohol. It has been proposed that the first stage in recovery from problem drinking is the recognition that the drinking is, indeed, problematic. This may happen gradually or as a result of some dramatic event (Saunders and Tate, 1983). A second stage involves the maintenance of the resolution to change and appears to be related to the ability and opportunity to change within the existing life style. Saunders and Kershaw (1979) found that a change in drinking habits was often sustained by the forming of new relationships, change of job, marriage or the onset of ill health, and Tuchfeld (1981) similarly found that the maintenance of behavioural changes was characterized by alterations in social, leisure and occupational activities. Drew (1968) suggested that the decreasing prevalence of heavy drinking with age is, in part, due to a spontaneous decrease associated with such factors.

Winnick (1962) has described the 'maturing out' of drug addicts, with the average length of 'addiction' being 8 to 10 years, and the majority giving up in their late twenties and early thirties. A follow-up of heroin 'addicts' in London suggested that about one-third had given up, about half of these without treatment or help (Wille, 1978). The giving up of heroin by Vietnam veterans on return to the USA has been documented by Robins et al., (1977).

The overall picture from such reports is of a substantial amount of self-initiated change, concomitant upon some meaningful event or change in personal circumstances. The initial impetus to change seems to be an external event which is integrated into the context of the individual's daily life.

Incidentally, it is interesting to speculate briefly on the doubt that such findings cast upon the whole notion of addiction. Smoking, alcohol abuse, drug-taking and overeating have all been labelled as addictions (Miller, 1980). However, it could be argued that this labeling process is carried out in the service of vested interests, by carrying the corollary that 'addictions' require professional treatment. Weiner (1980) has given an account of this management and marketing of social phenomena in her book on alcoholism.

The assumption that persistence with cigarette-smokng is due to physiological addiction is not necessarily sound. It has never been conclusively shown that nicotine produces dependency (McMorrow and Fox, 1983) and certainly some authors prefer to regard it as a consequence of very frequently repeated acts culminating in an entrenched habit (Hunt et al., 1967).

Studies of spontaneous smoking cessation have suggested that those who stop smoking on their own initiative go through a series of stages which begin with a gradual tendency to evaluate smoking and its effects (Prochaska and Di Clemente, 1982). Once in this 'contemplation' phase, smokers become more open to information and education about smoking and people report thinking more about themselves as smokers. This continuing evaluation is then inclined to lead to more attempts to stop (Prochaska and Di Clemente, 1983). It has been suggested that it is some combination of cognitive and affective processes which moves the person from contemplation to action. However, factors which move individuals into the contemplation stage have not been examined.

In-depth interviews carried out with people who had successfully changed some aspect of health related behaviour indicated that most changes were linked to circumstances which led people to reconsider some formerly habitual activity. The most important factors in leading people to contemplate change were difficulties with money, changing their social milieu so that certain behaviours became problematic (especially smoking and food habits) and changes in the structure of family life. Rarely were such changes a consequence of a concern with health (Hunt and MacLeod, 1987).

Studies of compliance with medical advice following diagnosis of a serious condition have indicated varying degrees of behavioural change from zero to the maximum suggested. A medical diagnosis or illness episode alone may bring about a certain amount of change. For example, a myocardial infarction or a diagnosis of angina has been found to be a strong predictor of smoking cessation (Weinblatt *et al.*, 1971). On the other hand, studies of people with chronic bronchitis and asthma have shown that many patients continue to smoke even in the face of severe exacerbation of symptoms (Nelson and Crofton, 1965; Kaptein, 1984).

A series of investigations carried out under the aegis of the National Heart, Lung and Blood Institute in the USA have suggested that several factors are implicated in improving compliance with recommendations of changes in health-related activities. These are: the frequency and continuity of contact with the doctor – greater where regular contact is provided (McGill, 1978); active participation by the patient in setting goals for changes in behaviour (Syme, 1976); social support and self-monitoring by the patient in the form of record-keeping with immediate direct feedback, e.g. changes in blood pressure levels can be related by the patient to actual behaviours (Earp and Ory, 1978; Kirscht and Rosenstock, 1977).

Research carried out in Canada has shown that training in first aid techniques is associated with safer driving behaviour and a reduction in road traffic accident rates (Miller and Agnew, 1973; Hunt, 1977). A prospective study by McKenna and Hale (1982) found that although workers who attended a 4 hour training course on emergency first aid had had a worse accident record than a matched control group prior to training, they manifested a significant reduction in accident injuries after training. The authors suggest that this may have been related to increased motivation to avoid accidents.

Another study assessed the effect of first aid training in a community on the accident injury rates in that community. The number of accident injuries to residents dropped significantly in a 26-month period following the training as compared with the rest of the country. Ruling out alternative explanations of the results, the most likely influence appeared to be the training itself. The authors carried out further investigations to try and ascertain the links between trainees and decreases in injury rates. It was found that volunteers for training were more likely than non-volunteers to be between 21 and 40 years of age; female; in employment; in contact with children of 15 years and under, both at home and at school. Surveys indicated that about 50 per cent of all trainees reported passing on information on first aid to family members, workmates and friends. It also seemed likely that there was a marked indirect effect whereby first aid trained parents influenced the environment and behaviour of their children so that they had fewer accident injuries, and there may have been a similar effect from teachers and others at school (Glendon and McKenna, 1985). What is particularly interesting about this research is that disaggregated data showed that accident injuries decreased significantly at home, school and work, where one would expect effects to be greatest, but not in the street or during leisure activities where the opportunity for direct and indirect influence is much less.

There have also been suggestions from workers in the USA that training of lay people in cardiopulmonary resuscitation (CPR) affects the health-related behaviour of trainees and their families and friends, although this evidence is largely anecdotal. The claim has been made that CPR education has played a role in lowering the cardiac death rate by creating recognition of cardiac emergencies as well as by teaching resuscitation, and has also helped in promoting healthier life styles by enhancing public awareness of risk factors in coronary heart disease. It seems that health-related training programmes, such as first aid and CPR, may have both direct and indirect effects which serve to give saliency to individual behaviour in a context which makes meaningful the possibility of change.

Drawing together the fragments of evidence from the wide variety of studies reported here it would seem that self-initiated behavioural change tends to occur when some formerly routine activity is brought into awareness for a prolonged period of time such that it becomes salient or problematic. This often takes place in conjunction with a change in the context in which the behaviour in question is being carried out, e.g. a smoker going to live with a non-smoker. The actions associated with a former 'habit' are now subject to cognitive appraisal, putting the individual in a situation where information about smoking, which was formerly filtered out, now impinges on perceptual processes. The presence and interest of significant others both provides reinforcement and helps to keep the behaviour in question salient. This approach suggests that changes in health-related behaviour take place as a consequence of a much more complex and meaningful set of processes than has hitherto been described.

The following formulation draws together empirical and theoretical material from a variety of disciplines in an attempt to construct a more holistic model of behavioural change in relation to health.

A Theory of Health-Related Behavioural Change

It should be emphasized that the theory to be outlined below is in its infancy and hypothesis-testing has only just begun. The content grew out of an attempt to integrate empirical data and explanatory propositions from a variety of disciplines. Expositions having the status of true theory are rare in health research and there is a need for firm theoretical foundations upon which to base strategies for improvements in health. The following should be viewed as a small step in this direction with an heuristic rather than a didactic intention.

Behaviour may be defined as combinations of individual acts which form patterns relatively peculiar to the individual, although such patterns may have a superficial similarity as a consequence of structural constraints. Behaviour patterns can be seen to fall into several categories: habitual routines e.g. brushing the teeth; environmentally constrained complex patterns, e.g. aspects of work; personal preferences, e.g. playing tennis; the relatively novel, new experiences which are a consequence of changed environment; impulse.

Taking the examples of smoking, alcohol use, eating and exercise, such behaviours may reasonably be supposed to be built into the flow of everyday life in a largely routine way; indeed they tend, for the most part, to fall into predictable and relatively stable patterns for any given individual. Such activities, therefore, are not normally subjected to much contemplation, coming to the forefront of consciousness only occasionally and then only in the most cursory way. They do not 'stand out' from on-going activities but are, rather, merely pointers in a continual and continuous series of interactions between the person, physiological and psychological processes, the outside environment and other people.

The genesis of habitual behaviour normally lies in the experience of a novel event or activity which, with repetition, loses its curiosity value, becomes overlearned with frequency and eventually is embedded in customary patterns of activity. Thus, during the acquisition of a habit there is participation at the highest level of cognitive processing in the brain, involving cerebral activity and cellular changes which are the physical components of learning. After the formation of a habit or skill, high-level participation is no longer necessary and the activity may come to depend upon a different and lower-level set of zones in the brain (Luria et al., 1970). Habitual activities are probably regulated by the medial regions of the cortex, above the upper brain stem and reticular formation (MacLean, 1959). It has been demonstrated that lesions in these areas lead to the disruption of habitual activities in human beings (Luria, 1973). Such activities are, therefore, carried out with a minimum of awareness, coming to the forefront of consciousness only briefly at time intervals of varying length. An example of this change in the level of processing is the transition from being a learner to becoming an experienced car driver. Initially, the individual acts which make up the behaviour of driving must receive total attention and concentration. The more often the sequences of acts are performed the more routine and 'natural' they become, until eventually a minimum of awareness accompanies the behaviour involved in driving and long periods of time may pass without any clear consciousness of the activities being performed. Miller, Galanter and Pribram (1965) refer to the PLAN, i.e. a series of actions incorporated into a hierarchical process. Habits and skills are at the lower end of the hierarchy and acts which were once voluntary become relatively inflexible and fixed by overlearning.

This notion of a hierarchical organization of physiological and psychological processes is also present in linguistic theory (Carroll, 1953), and in studies of animal behaviour (Tinbergen, 1951). Several psychologists have echoed this theme. Allport (1961) used the term 'functional autonomy' to describe habitual behaviours; Hunt and Matarazzo (1970) have written of the 'habitual, affectless' behaviour which has, 'the blandness of habit' and Kelly (1955) commented on the lack of conscious thought about behaviour specifically in relation to gambling, alcohol use and sex.

The relegation of habits to lower levels of consciousness may be seen as part of a general adaptation process which allows the person to deal with a potentially huge number of internal and external events and the information contained within them when 'channel capacity' is limited. In this way higher-level monitoring and decision-making processes are free to deal with the more novel and salient features of daily life.

It is only when some relatively novel event occurs, requiring special attention, that descending messages from the cortex re-arouse awareness of some aspect of the habit. This appears to be part of the function of the reticular formation of the brain which influences perception and the focus of concentration by its 'pattern matching' processes; that is, relatively common, routine stimuli are often filtered out and preference is given to the relatively novel stimuli whether they arise internally or externally.

The relegation of the mundane to lower levels frees the person to concentrate on more complex and comparatively 'difficult' activities (Luria et al., 1970). Such processes have also been expressed in the epistemology of Piaget (1936) where they have been described, albeit in very different language, as comprising part of the adaptational dynamic which keeps a person in equilibrium, in constant interaction with new elements in the environment, whilst incorporated knowledge becomes deeply embedded.

From a phenomenological point of view it has been argued that human beings live simultaneously in various realms of reality with varying degrees of attention to the inner world of thought and experience and the outer world of phenomena, Schutz (1970) uses the phrase 'counterpointal personality' (analogous to independent themes in a piece of music) to describe the ability to attend to one theme out of two or more which are coterminous. According to Schutz only very superficial levels of the self are involved in habitual acts and 'quasi-automatic' chores such as eating or dressing. It may be postulated that cigarette-smoking and alcohol use also have this quasi-automatic' quality where they are indulged in on a regular basis.

In the world of routine activities much is taken for granted as 'typical situations' and 'typical interactions' are encountered and we follow routines as long as nothing arises which might interfere with the usual processes of everyday life. Schutz (1970) refers to 'topics-in-hand' as having lost their 'interpretational relevance'. That is, familiar acts no longer arouse our curiosity. 'They have become slotted into the stream of daily life. Yet. . . . if something hampers the on going routine, action, the topic-in-hand prevailing up to then may go 'out of hand' and the topic may become again a theme and all its horizons again open to interpretational questioning.' (p. 140)

The drawing together of this physiological, psychological and sociological material does cast light on the nature of some health-related activities. Although for health educators, smoking, alcohol use, exercise and diet may be highly salient, forming the focus of daily thought and activity, for the actors these behaviours are 'routine' performed at lower levels of brain functioning and subjected to minimum thought and attention. The lack of salience of such behaviours has important implications for the perceptual processes of the individuals concerned. In the course of waking life, myriad sights, sounds, smells and other stimuli present possibilities for attention. Perception of a selection of these stimuli is not a passive process, whereby an individual sees, hears or smells whatever is within perceptual distance. He or she may be exposed to many things, but relatively few reach the level of conscious attention. Perception is the end-product of a comparison and/or a summation which takes place between incoming information and internal processes (Gyr Brown et al., 1966). Since not everything can be attended to 'choices' are made. 'Thus what is seen or heard tends to be that which is of interest, relevance or importance to the individual (Neisser, 1976). This selection procedure will, naturally, be related to the context and meaning of the events and messages available. Thus, we may deduce that selective perception processes will ensure that although health 'messages may be vaguely seen, they are not topics for attention unless the routine behaviour in question has already become salient for some other reason.

Occasionally, individuals will be confronted with some piece of information which it is impossible for them to 'choose' not to attend to, as might be the case, for example, with advice to stop smoking being given by a doctor to a person who has suffered a heart attack.

Faced with information which stresses the importance and utility of change, many individuals still decide to ignore what appears to be excellent, even life-enhancing and life-preserving advice. Two notions are of relevance here: that of 'reactance (Brehm, 1966) and that of 'containment' (Goffman, 1963; Alonzo, 1984).

Studies of 'reactance' have shown that people often react adversely to what they perceive as attempts to restrict their freedom of choice. Thus a person who has in his or her repertoire a certain type of behaviour which is perceived to be under attack will exhibit reactance. It is said that the greater the perceived threat, the greater the reaction against it. The importance of the behaviour to the individual and the extent to which there is a strongly felt need to indulge in the behaviour will also influence the arousal and the extent of reactance. Thus, telling someone he or she must take more exercise may be interpreted as an attack on the freedom to be slothful and will merely confirm or even strengthen sedentary tendencies (Brehm, 1966).

The concept of 'containment' rests upon the interactionist view of the social world as inherently unstable and, therefore, requiring a continual set of adaptational responses to environmental contingencies, both social and physical (Mead, 1934; Cooley, 1902). The necessity for constant adaptation imposes a strain on the coping abilities of the individual as he, or she, attempts to maintain a stable perspective. A certain set about the self and the external world is developed with which the individual is, in some sense, comfortable. Any situation encountered by an individual is said to have both 'performance' aspects, in terms of the skills, capacities and resources it may require, and 'impact' aspects which refer to the consequences for the individual of being in that situation. Containment refers to an individual's tendency to refrain from becoming more than minimally affected by situations which are perceived as too demanding. Containment will be affected by the individual's commitment to certain behaviours, beliefs, goals and so on which form part of self-identity; by the availability of resources, social, psychological or financial; by issues of social propriety, that is, the extent to which others would comment, and by the need to maintain a particular role performance.

Attempts to change routine behaviours related to health may confront containment processes and threaten social and psychological integrity by bringing certain issues into the foreground in a manner which threatens adaptational resources. Resistance will, therefore, be aroused, one form of which may be to 'refuse' to allow certain subjects to become the focus of attention. This is particularly likely to be the case where individuals are already in situations which heavily tax their coping ability.

Prerequisites for change

Using the foregoing information as a framework, it should be possible to specify the minimum conditions under which changes of health-related behaviour are most likely to take place. Beginning with the premise that the four health-related behaviours under consideration have a routine nature, it is assumed that these do not normally engage attentional processes beyond the minimum necessary for the performance of the acts of which they are made up. Such behaviours are originally adopted with full awareness, but with familiarity and constant repetition gradually fall below the level of conscious attention. The first prerequisite for change is, therefore, that the behaviour should again become salient and, therefore, be subjected to scrutiny in the context of on-going everyday life. Secondly, the way in which this occurs should not be so direct as to result in reactance or to confront containment processes. Thirdly, the behaviour should remain under cognitive appraisal over a period of time. Fourthly, change will be more likely to occur where adaptational processes are not already under strain. Fifthly, the 'climate of opinion' should be such that changes in selective attention concomitant upon some behaviour becoming problematic will provide information about the desirability and direction of any change There must be opportunity to change the behaviour in question and, finally, behaviour will be least likely to change where it plays a role in important coping strategies. For example, it has been pointed out that 'drugs of solace' play a significant part in adaptational processes by alleviating distress and providing psychological and social comfort (Cameron and Jones, 1985). Some empirical support for this theory is available, e.g. the studies of changes in behaviour subsequent to first aid training are clearly compatible with such a formulation.

The routinized orientation of medical specialists to clinical decision-making has been described by Bloor (1978) who suggested that the treatment of patients does not arise from some reasoned calculation about the relative suitability of the available therapeutic procedures, but rather emerges 'automatically' from a set of 'routine decision rules' which remain cognitively unexamined. Other authors have described similar processes in the decision-making of coroners (Atkinson, 1971), hospital staff (Sudnow, 1967) and general practitioners (Fletcher, 1974).

A study by Hunt et al. (1987) demonstrated how this routinization can be interrupted. During the course of involvement in an investigation of prescribing habits in a general practice, doctors became aware of problematic aspects of their prescriptions, primarily cost and failure to choose generic drugs when available. The context of the exercise was familiar, the material meaningful and the opportunity for change available. Subsequently, prescribing behaviour was modified.

A specific test of the theory has also been carried out in relation to food habits. This involved the recruitment and training of a group of paid volunteers from a small community in Scotland to carry out a survey of food habits. The rationale was that the training procedures and the survey would have the effect of making routine behaviour salient and retaining that salience for a period of time within a meaningful context. A cross-over design with a study in a similar area was utilized to provide a quasi-control group. The main hypothesis was that the experimental group, that is, the group carrying out the food survey, would exhibit significant behavioural change in relation to their own food habits as compared with the control group.

After the survey had been completed, it was established that there were significant differences between the experimental and control groups in relation to key behaviours, with over half of the experimental group exhibiting some change whilst there was none in the control group. In spite of a number of problems, which principally arose because of the 'naturalistic' research design used, the results from this preliminary test, although extremely modest, provide some support for the proposed theory of behavioural change Hunt and Martin (1988). One problem associated with the way in which subjects were recruited relates to possible 'volunteer effects'. However, as everyone was volunteering for paid work, not dietary modification, it is unlikely that this would have affected the results. A further possibility is that the observed changes in behaviour were due to the demand characteristics of the task. However, there were a considerable number of areas in which change in the 'desired' direction could have occurred – consumption of cereal, pulses, vegetables, etc.- but the only real differences found were in relation to the kind of bread eaten. Moreover, for almost all of the many variables studied there was remarkable consistency in the pattern of responses for each subject from the first to the second administration of the questionnaire. This, in turn, suggests that the reported behaviours were genuine reports of actual behaviours and that the reported changes were genuine ones. Further tests of hypotheses arising from the study are currently under way.

Training procedures are just one way of inducing involvement in a particular issue, but they do provide the essential elements of raising hitherto routine issues, learning in a meaningful context, having the opportunity to fit the knowledge gained into existing schemata, being able to apply the knowledge in a familiar social context and the discussion of implications with significant others. It seems reasonable to assume that change growing out of some 'natural' cognitive reorganization on the part of the subject will be longer lasting than that which is, as it were, imposed artificially from without.

This approach implies that behaviour can be adequately explained only by taking into account the context in which it occurs (Strauss, 1981). Thus theories of behavioural change and attempts to influence behaviour must take account of the social setting in which individuals carry out the behaviours in question.

Discussion

A common means of gathering baseline data is to ask people if and why they carry out certain health-related behaviours, with the underlying assumption that the behaviours in question are the subject of deep cogitation by the people concerned. It is possible that this represents a misleading categorization of routine behaviours as conscious behaviours through the activity of asking questions. When asked about their 'attitude' to, say, alcohol use, people will generally give an answer which appears to be a justification for their behaviour which has an a priori character. However, the model presented here focuses rather on the proposition put forward by Schutz that actions are defined through meaning and that the stream of consciousness has no intrinsic meaning. It is only once an experience has passed that it can be lifted out of the 'stream' to become a 'thing' that can be assigned a meaning. Thus, experience is grasped only in retrospect. At the time of its occurrence, behaviour is a 'pre-phenomenal' experience. It is the 'backward glance' of reflection that endows significance (Schutz, 1972). Thus, many actions flow along in a largely unregarded manner, but if a person is forced to reflect on these actions, e.g. by being asked a question about them, some post hoc justification will be given, the content of which may well be related more to the context of the inquiry than to some 'true' description.

The theory presented here gives rise to several testable postulates, of which a few are described below.

1. Individual change is initiated by some event or activity which raises some behaviour to a level which causes it to be subjected to cognitive appraisal, by lifting it out of 'the stream of consciousness'. Research currently being carried out at RUHBC suggests that three types of initiation of change exist: 'traumatic', that is, when a sudden event brings certain health-related behaviours into focus, e.g. the death of a loved one, illness, loss of a job; 'socio environmental'. when because of a change in social circumstances some behaviour becomes problematic, e.g. a meat-eater sharing a flat with a group of vegetarians; and 'cognitive', that is, a long process of consideration of some behaviour and a weighing of the pros and cons of changing it. This latter approximates most closely to the 'rational' approach.

2. The new salience of a behaviour brings about changes in selective perception such that formerly unnoticed aspects of the world come into focus. However, in order for change to occur this change in perception must be prolonged; hence the efficacy

of carrying out some task related to the behaviour in question, as in the survey of food habits, first aid and CPR training. Other studies have also stressed the importance of involvement in some relevant activity as being related to subsequent change, e.g. Cartwright (1949); and Bandura (1979). Studies of behaviour modification which use cognitive restructuring have used internal 'monologues' associated with undesirable habits which prevent the habits from returning to the routine level by constantly reiterating statements which are incompatible with the behaviour in question (Lazarus, 1971; Ziesat, 1977).

3. Changes in behaviour will be difficult to maintain unless and until the new behaviour (which may, of course, be the non-performing of the old behaviour) becomes relegated also to the routine level of physiological and cognitive processing. This point was made many years ago by William James (1891) that new habits must become firmly rooted in daily life before successful change could occur. One of the reasons why, for example, smokers are in danger of relapse may be that not smoking is problematic and, therefore, remains as a conscious issue. Nisbett (1972) has pointed out that people who have a problem with food intake and who are often on diets restrict their food intake by conscious cognitive self-control – 'high-restraint' eaters. 'Low restraint' eaters conversely, never give much consideration to what they eat. It is the 'high-restraint' eaters who are most susceptible to relapse (Herman and Mack, 1975) again perhaps because the new diet is never allowed to become a habit through the relinquishing of awareness.

4. Some changes will be easier than others. Qualitative changes, say from white bread to wholemeal, should be the easiest because the new behaviour is very close to the old. On the other hand, giving something up, e.g. cigarettes, should be the most difficult unless substitute activities can be found (which themselves may not be particularly healthy, e.g. some women prefer to smoke rather than substitute eating (Hunt and McLeod, 1987)). Taking up an activity, such as exercise, will require sufficient repetition for it to become habitual and will thus be susceptible to failure unless prolonged. For this reason it is probably easier to maintain exercise when it is built into the flow of everyday life – e.g. walking to work rather than driving – rather than being 'artificially' tacked on – e.g. going to 'keep fit' classes.

5. Individuals whose lives involve many problems, and high uncertainty and whose coping strategies and resources are limited will be least likely to change behaviours. The often noted intransigence of disadvantaged socioeconomic groups in relation to heeding health advice could be because their adaptive energies are already fully taxed by trying to get by on a low income, living in poor housing, having children who are more likely to get sick, being unemployed, and so on. In addition, where change is attempted maintenance will be more difficult. In such cases, therefore, the most efficacious strategy will be to ameliorate the conditions of deprivation and disadvantage rather than to subject the victims of such circumstances to further strain.

6. Change will not take place unless the opportunity is available, e.g. an ability to obtain and afford fresh fruit.

For some of these postulates evidence already exists, others are in the process of being tested and the remainder await suitable investigation.

Conclusions

Changes in public health which require alteration or modification of individual habits will only be brought about through understanding the nature and context of human behaviour. Whilst health education and health promotion may provide an outside climate which influences the direction and content of behavioural changes they are unlikely to trigger such changes while still based upon the 'rational' approach. The most efficacious, practical and hopeful of current initiatives in health, on the basis of the model presented here, is probably community development. Only when people's lives become less strained and adaptive processes are relatively untaxed will they be likely to consider changes in basic behaviours.

The community development approach of involving local people in health issues and encouraging participation in decision-making and strategies for social change, is not only more humanitarian but is also more likely to result in change, not as a consequence of direct confrontation of 'unhealthy habits' but rather as a result of such habits slowly being subjected to cognitive appraisal. These processes will also occur within a context which is meaningful and supportive.

Hitherto, community development strategies have lacked a sound theoretical basis. It is hoped that the refinement and development of the model presented here will help provide such a foundation.

CHAPTER 6

Disadvantage and Disease

The most constantly observed characteristic of the patterning of the incidence and prevalence of disease in populations is of a gradient in morbidity and mortality rates which is closely linked to social class. People in the lower socioeconomic groupings suffer a disproportionate amount of disease and disability and have a curtailed longevity. Antonovsky (1967) in a review of the literature remarked that this association had been known since as far back as the twelfth century.

The publication of the *Black Report* in Britain drew attention yet again to the accumulated evidence that the gap in health status between the more and the less affluent members of society was becoming wider (DHSS, 1980) in spite of a National Health Service, the avowed intention of which was to 'divorce health care from personal finance or other factors irrelevant to health' (HMSO, 1944). More recently a report on health inequalities in the 1980s – *The Health Divide* – has indicated that in the last 8 years this gap has become even wider (Whitehead, 1987). The association between social class and risks to health is very close, not only in Great Britain but also in other countries where such information is reliably and routinely collected. While it is true that mortality has declined somewhat for the poor, there has been an even greater decline for the better-off. In earlier years differences in death rates from infectious diseases and infant mortality rates linked to poor hygiene, overcrowding and deficient antenatal and postnatal care probably accounted for a large proportion of the social class differentials. Current differences, however, must be attributed primarily, although not wholly, to non-infectious conditions.

In Britain, the *General Household Survey* (OPCS, 1978) indicated that men and women from lower social classes report higher rates of both chronic and acute illness and tend to consult their family doctor more often than do the higher classes. This class differential becomes less steep with age as the likelihood of death increases. For example, among males aged under 44 years, the ratio of deaths between social class V and social class I is 2.45, falling to 1.7 at 45 years and over. The risk of death before retirement in both sexes is two and a half times as great in unskilled manual workers and their wives as it is in professional men and their wives. The relationship between social class and morbidity does not appear to hold true for women aged 15 to 44 years, perhaps because of the convention of classifying married women by their husband's occupation.

General hospital acute beds are used more by lower social classes and they stay in hospital longer (Cartwright and Paterson, 1966). This may be related to poor housing conditions and adverse domestic circumstances as well as possibly longer recovery rates. Although classes IV and V represent 21% and 9% respectively of the population, they account for 26.5% and 14.2% of hospital beds occupied (Ministry of Health, 1967). Even so, it has been concluded that the hospitalization rates of this group are less than would be expected from their experience of ill health and probable need for care (Abel-Smith and Titmuss, 1956; Alderson, 1966).

In addition to morbidity and mortality differentials, there are also class gradients in height, weight, birth weight, eye defects and dental health (Brotherston, 1976). These associations between social class and health indicators have been observed in countries as diverse as the USA (Syme and Berkman, 1976), Finland (Naytia, 1977), Australia (Nixon and Pearn, 1980) and France (Derrienec, 1977).

In spite of the consistency and ubiquity of these findings, the use of social class as an indicator of social disadvantage has come in for much criticism. Jones and Cameron (1984) have described it as deriving from '. . . an empiricist methodology which has been engineered to conform to the prejudices of narrow-minded professionals' (p. 37).

They point out that classifications are closely related to educational and informational requirements of occupations. It is, therefore, scarcely surprising that other aspects of social structure which are also related to education, like health, should be associated with social class. Moreover, social class gradients conceal wide variations in mortality within social classes. Standardized mortality rates in social class I range from 42 for electrical engineers to 116 for pharmacists and, within social class V, from 80 for builders' labourers to 160 for engineering labourers. The applicability of the classifications to women is also quite equivocal.

It is clear, then, that social class, although perhaps useful as a starting-point, is too global and ambiguous a categorization to be of much heuristic value in explaining differences in health status between groups. Skrimshire (1978) found, for example, that sickness rates in young people were higher in a deprived than a non-deprived area with a similar working-class population. Brotherston (1976) pointed out that the health experiences of people in social class I living in a poor area are close to those of people in social class Ill who live in affluent areas. A study in Newcastle found that differences in health status within social class Ill were as wide as those between social classes I and V (Neligman et al. 1974). Nevertheless, the consistency with which social class is linked to disability and disease, in spite of differences in ways of calculating it, uncertainties of classification and cultural diversity, has given rise to a number of attempts to explain the observed data.

Explanations of Social Class Differences

Access to health care

A principal aim of the National Health Service was to provide access to health care for all sections of the population. There is considerable debate about how far this has been achieved. Tudor-Hart (1971), for example, has argued that health care is actually superior in areas of low need and, conversely, tends to be poor in areas of high need. It has also been suggested that the middle classes make more efficient and effective use of health services than do less well-educated and linguistically skilled groups (Titmuss, 1968; Cartwright and O'Brien, 1976.) Important issues are whether:

—provision is unequal
—access is unequal, or
—inequalities in access and/or provision contribute to health inequalities.

Since more deprived communities have poorer health they do, theoretically, have a greater need for health care (Backett, 1977). An analysis of *General Household Survey* data indicated that, contrary to the findings of some other studies, there was no bias against lower socioeconomic groups in access to primary care facilities and that, moreover, rates of utilization for some disease categories were proportionately higher than rates of self-reported morbidity would indicate (Collins and Klein, 1980). The validity of these conclusions, where 'need' could not be matched with 'use' for individuals and where frequency of use was not standardized for different categories of health need and socioeconomic status, has been criticized by Scott-Samuel (1981). Consultation rates in lower socioeconomic groups do not appear to match morbidity experience. Boucquet and Curtis (1986) found that the higher levels of distress in feelings of fatigue, sleep disturbance, pain and emotional problems for manual groups were not matched by differential use of health services.

The Black Report (DHSS, 1980) concluded that, for the most part, class differences in ill health were not matched by class differences in utilization rates. There is, however, some evidence that men in social class V in the 15–64 age group make greater use of out-patient services than males in other groups. In-patient data from Scottish hospitals show a clear gradient, with men and, less markedly, women in the lower social classes having higher hospitalization rates. This pattern also holds for children. People in social classes IV and V are not only hospitalized more often than would be expected but also tend to stay longer once they are there (Carstairs and Paterson, 1966). A report comparing death and discharge rates with social indicators in Camberwell wards showed that both paediatric and geriatric hospitalization rates and length of stay varied directly by indices of social deprivation, as did length of stay in the maternity unit (Hunt, 1984).

The somewhat patchy evidence which aggregates and, thus, largely obscures the reasons behind these patterns suggests that, although greater health needs are not always matched by higher consultation and hospitalization rates, those individuals in the lower occupational groupings tend to make more use of health services for treatment purposes. However, since these groups also have greater needs, differences in consultation rates alone cannot contribute to the initial health inequalities.

Two aspects of health service use, nevertheless, interact with and may exacerbate inequalities between social classes: quality of care and use of preventive services. Pendleton and Bochner (1980) found that the level of spontaneously proffered information and explanation given by general practitioners was greater for middle-class as compared to working-class patients. Similarly, middle-class patients may make better use of consultation time in terms of the information which is sought and offered (Cartwright and O'Brien, 1976). Socially, educationally and linguistically middle-class patients have more in common with their doctors than do working-class patients and this, in turn, creates advantages for the former in medical encounters. The desire for information is, however, no different between the two types of patients (Cartwright and Anderson, 1981).

Working-class women appear to make less use of a wide range of preventive services and the effects of this are compounded by a greater prevalence of potentially preventable or treatable disorders in that group. Thus, mortality may be even greater than would be expected on the basis of numbers at risk alone. Middle-class women have a higher risk of breast cancer, possibly because of their tendency to later child-bearing, but they also manifest a greater use of screening services (Van den Heuvel, 1978). This tends to undermine the argument that inequalities in morbidity and mortality can be accounted for by under-use of preventive services. In addition, since only a limited number of conditions actually are preventable the most that can be hoped for from screening is early detection and treatment.

At a more global level it is unlikely that differential use of health facilities could account for more than a small proportion of social class differences in health, simply because of the limited impact of health services on the health of the population as compared to social conditions and public health measures (McKeown, 1980).

Artefact explanations

It has been suggested that the observed relationship between social class and mortality rates is no more than an artefact arising from systematic error in the way in which data are collected and classified (Stern, 1983). For example, under the classificatory system of the Registrar-General, individuals with irregular working experiences and those who are difficult to classify may be assigned to lower social classes. Moreover, revisions made in the categorizaton of occupations may render strict comparisons invalid. The assignment of occupations to classes is subject to change and the relative size of classes has changed over the years since the system was introduced. The number of people in the two lower social classes is much smaller than it was 50 years ago (Registrar General, 1978). Occupational mortality statistics tend to be subject to bias in both numerator and denominator because of discrepancies between occupations reported in the Census and those reported at death. However, the differential in mortality between the highest and the lowest social class is rather too extreme to be accounted for by misclassifications, and death certificates have been found to be of reasonable accuracy in respect of previous occupation (Heasman and Lipworth, 1969). Moreover, analyses by Koskinen (1985) taking artefact effects into account still indicated a widening in class differences in mortality since 1951. This was confirmed in the work of Pamuk (1985), who also showed that changes in classification had little effect on mortality trends.

Social mobility

Another explanation of social class differences in health has been that they are largely due to the fact that unhealthy individuals, particularly those with long-standing chronic disorders, are likely to 'drift' down the social ladder and die in a lower social class than the one they started off in, thus making the mortality rates of the lowest socioeconomic grouping artificially high. Related to this is the argument that very healthy people are likely to move in the opposite direction (Stern, 1983; Lawrence, 1958). Alternatively, as Harkey *et al.* (1976) have argued, poor health may act as a barrier to upward social mobility and those who function well on a consistent basis will slowly tend to become better-off and their children will move up the social scale. In their study, an excess of disease and disability in 25–34-year-olds in the lowest social classes could have been, in part, attributable to downward social drift, but a greater amount of the variance was, in fact, accounted for by movement out of the lowest income groups by healthier persons.

Illsley (1955, 1967) suggested that taller and healthier women were more likely to marry upward socially, whilst the reverse would be the case for smaller and less healthy women. Thus, the upper social echelons are reinforced with the 'best' of the stock from the lower and the obverse phenomenon occurs at the other end of the scale. Furthermore, this creates a wide gap between extremes in terms of the probability of their mating (or even meeting, presumably) because of their different health experiences.

The social class gradient in chronic bronchitis has been attributed to downward mobility (Meadows, 1963). A similar argument has been put forward for schizophrenia by Goldberg and Morrison (1963) who showed that the fathers of patients had a higher social class, on average, than their offspring. However, an analysis of mortality rates in the period 1976–81 in England and Wales among a 1% sample of the Census who are being studied longitudinally, indicated that mortality gradients at ages after retirement were almost as steep as those found in the later stages of working life (Fox *et al.*, 1985). At ages over 75 years, men in social class V had mortality rates 50% higher than those in social class 1. A social drift hypothesis could scarcely encompass differentials in those oldest age groups, since the men concerned had probably been retired for 10 years or more. This analysis also demonstrated that the mortality gradient by social class 5 to 10 years before death is very close to that pertaining at the time of death, thus indicating that health-related social mobility is unlikely to be more than a minor factor in social class differences.

Blane (1985) has argued strongly against the social drift explanation on the grounds that studies of specific populations, such as those of Goldberg and Morrison (1963) and Meadows (1963), have been unrepresentative, generally exclusive of women and/ or largely confined to hospital patients. He points out that many diseases such as cardiovascular and gastrointestinal disorders, as well as respiratory complaints (other than bronchitis), do not appear to show social mobility effects. He also makes the point that if social drift were a common phenomenon, diseases which are quickly fatal – e.g. lung cancer – would be expected to show less steep gradients than would slow degenerative conditions like chronic bronchitis. This, however, is not the case, the two conditions showing rather similar gradients with social class.

Hunt *et al.* (1985) found that differences in perceived health status, particularly in relation to emotional problems, sleep and feelings of fatigue, were related to social class only in younger age groups well before social drift could be expected to occur. This would seem to argue for pre-existing distress in social classes IV and V. A recent analysis by Alexander *et al.* (1987) demonstrates a very high association between area of residence and mortality rates in women aged 45–64 years. The more social indicators of deprivation in an area the higher the mortality from all causes. Since the vast majority of these women are married, a social drift hypothesis would appear to be disconfirmed unless their husbands are drifting down the social scale simultaneously.

Constitutional-social hypotheses

A more complex approach to explaining the association between social class and ill health brings together a number of interacting biological and social events which are said to be responsible both for the causation and the perpetuation of the phenomenon.

Baird (1975) presented data which suggested differential reproductive ability in relation to maternal height and physique and hypothesized that early social deprivation affected the constitution and reproductive efficiency of the offspring. Illsley (1986) compared the percentage of mothers over 5 feet 4 inches tall in social classes I and II with the percentage in social classes IV and V. The difference between these groups was 15.2% classifying by father's occupation and 18.3% classifying by husband's occupation – an increase of 20% in the height differential. Perinatal mortality rates in the two groupings increased by 116% when women were reclassified from their family of origin to their family of marriage. Baird (1974) has also argued that the female children of women who were themselves deprived tend to suffer the effects of damage inflicted on their mothers or of deleterious behaviours in their mothers, which are in turn compounded by their own adverse social circumstances.

It is assumed that a poor economic, social and physical environment exacerbates constitutional and genetic weaknesses, so that when children from the lower social classes grow up they have few skills and little opportunity to succeed occupationally. The work they do do, if indeed they find work at all, will tend to be unrewarding, stressful, of uncertain stability and, of course, low paid (Illsley, 1980). This 'cycle of deprivation' model suggests that the life pattern of a child is largely determined before its birth (Davie *et al.*, 1972) and tends to assume that there is a constant pool of biological and social 'weaklings' which is in some sense self-perpetuating.

There is support for this view in so far as children from deprived backgrounds do tend to be of short stature, to underachieve in school and to go on to low-paid work in unskilled jobs (Blaxter, 1981). However, Goldthorpe (1980) has shown evidence for considerable social mobility and a major proportion of people in the higher social classes come from families which, at some time in their fairly recent history, came from the lower classes. The work of Blaxter and Paterson (1982) in Aberdeen suggests that subsequent generations, even lacking a decent education, are better informed than previous ones and that the problems they face are of a different nature. Aspects of deprivation may be constant, but they are not stagnant. Wilkinson (1986) has cast doubt on the data presented by Illsley by pointing out that since estimates of inter-and intra-generational mobility depend upon comparing the social class of the reported occupation of two different people or of one person at two points in time respectively, the accuracy of the information will be affected by the extent and detail of the informant's knowledge. The informant may, for example, be able to remember that his or her father worked for the railways, but not in what capacity or whether skilled or unskilled.

Behavioural Explanations

In recent years the aetiology of the major causes of death has come to be associated with so-called 'risk factors', which have generally been defined to be a consequence of the behaviour of individuals. Thus, lung cancer, cardiovascular diseases and strokes have been attributed largely to cigarette-smoking, poor diet, lack of exercise and alcohol consumption, separately or in combination. This approach has a particular appeal to governments reluctant to engage in public spending, to a medical profession with an individualistic orientation and to health educators whose brief it is to eliminate 'ignorance' about the effects of behaviour on health status. The assumptions behind this view are twofold: that these behaviours are indeed major contributors to disease processes and, by implication, since the lower social classes suffer a disproportionate amount of such diseases, that they, as a subsection of society, are particularly likely to indulge in 'unhealthy' habits. Thus it would be expected that the behaviours in question should exhibit a similar social class gradient as do morbidity and mortality data.

Taking the four most commonly cited risk factors, that is, smoking, excessive alcohol consumption, diet and exercise, each will be examined in turn for its possible role in disease processes and its association, if any, with social class.

Smoking

It has been estimated that in the United Kingdom some 50,000 people die every year as a direct result of cigarette-smoking (Royal College of Physicians, 1977). Cigarettes have been linked to increased risk of a variety of cancers, including those of the lung, bladder, nose, throat and mouth and to coronary heart disease, cerebrovascular accidents, chronic obstructive airways disease and peripheral vascular disease, even though it is not always possible to disentangle effects due to smoking from those related to other factors. Infants of smoking mothers are more likely to be miscarried, to be underweight and to show excess mortality than are those of non-smokers (USDHEW, 1979). Inhalation of tobacco smoke in the environment by children aged under 1 year is said to constitute a risk to their health (Ferguson et al., 1981).

It has been said that the cessation of smoking alone would reduce mortality from all cancers by approximately one-third, from aortic aneurysm by three-quarters and from myocardial infarction by about a quarter (Doll, 1983), although the author does not speculate as to whether this would convey immortality on some people and, if not, what they could expect to die of instead.

According to the General Household Survey carried out in 1984, the proportion of men and women reporting that they had never smoked regularly is much higher in professional men and in non-manual workers and their spouses (OPCS, 1985). In 1972, nearly twice as many unskilled manual workers smoked as did professional men, although the differential was much less for women; 33% professional women as compared to 42% off unskilled women workers reported that they smoked. In the years between 1976 and 1984 a trend towards reduction in smoking was reported by all socioeconomic groups, except professionals.

However, of those who did smoke in 1972 and subsequent years, the actual number of cigarettes smoked per week was not very different between social classes. Moreover, for every year the heaviest smokers, both men and women, were from among the skilled not unskilled manual workers. Professional and managerial groups were the most likely to report having given up smoking (OPCS, 1985). However, there is some evidence that when social class is measured by a woman's own occupation, instead of that of her husband, there is a high proportion of regular smokers in the professional and managerial groups (Jacobson, 1981). Approximately 50% of nurses, for example, are estimated to be regular smokers (Medical News, 1983).

Smoking has been found to be more common in the children of manual workers irrespective of parental smoking (Bewley *et al.*, 1980) and Calnan and Rutter (1986) found smoking to be significantly more prevalent in working-class as compared to middle-class women in the age group 45 to 64 years. The evidence that smoking is linked to several diseases is irrefutable, although controversy exists about the nature of the link and its effects are likely to be compounded by other factors. The evidence for the concentration of smoking in the lowest social classes is more ambiguous.

Exercise

Low levels of strenuous physical activity are characteristic of the populations of western industrialized countries. This has been said to be a contributory factor in the causation of obesity, high blood pressure, adverse blood lipid levels and, by implication, athero-sclerosis (Leon *et al.*, 1979). Sedentary individuals who take up moderate exercise show improvement in oxygen transport and in muscle and cardiovascular functioning (Satin *et al.*, 1976; Hanson *et al.*, 1968). Programmes for weight reduction which include exercise as well as dietary control have been shown to be more successful than those which involve dietary restriction alone (Glick Kaufman, 1976; Sidney *et al.*, 1977). There appears to be evidence that vigorous exercise, whether in leisure or work activities, is linked to a lower incidence of coronary heart disease (Morris *et al.*, 1973; Paffenbarger and Hale, 1975) although it is difficult to separate the propensity to take exercise from other characteristics of the individual and the environment which might also be relevant. For example, the ability to engage in hard physical activity is itself dependent upon feelings of well-being. Exercise has been found to reduce blood pressure in hypertensives and to lower triglyceride levels and increase the proportion of high to low density lipoproteins (Bonano and Lies, 1974; Brunner *et al.*, 1977; Lewis *et al.*, 1976). Regular physical activity also seems to enhance mental health; people report that they feel better after physical exercise, they have a reduced sense of effort for physical tasks and apparently experience psychological benefits (Borg and Linderholm, 1975; Heinzelman and Bagley, 1970; Myrtek and Villinger, 1976).

People who live in low-income areas are much less likely to engage in organized sport such as tennis, squash or badminton, but they are more likely to play and watch football than people in higher income areas. Those who live in very deprived districts record very high scores on sedentary pursuits such as watching television and betting and very low scores on sporting activities and gardening (Shaw, 1984). Working-class women report taking less exercise than do women in higher income groups (Calnan and Rutter, 1986). Managers, professionals and non-manual workers have been found to be more active in their leisure time than blue-collar workers, possibly because they expend much less energy at work. However, definitions of 'active' vary widely and it is impossible to estimate whether individuals of higher socioeconomic status are more active to the extent that it benefits their health (Stephens *et al.*, 1985).

In general, however, regardless of income or disadvantage, the level of active partici-pation in sports and exercise is quite low in Britain and the overall percentage of the population who report taking regular exercise has, in fact, remained stable over the past 10 years.

Alcohol

The question of how much alcohol is too much has given rise to a variety of answers, the list of which will not be added to here. Excessive alcohol intake has been implicated in several disorders including chronic liver diseases, cirrhosis of the liver, pancreatic damage, gastrointestinal changes, heart disease, brain damage and, most recently, sexual dysfunction and changes in the sex organs (Royal College of Psychiatrists, 1986, 1987). The relationship between alcohol levels in drivers and accidents is well established (DOE, 1976). In addition, alcohol abuse is believed to lead to a variety of psychological and social problems, marital disharmony, job loss and crime (Heather *et al.*, 1985). In some cases, however, it may well be impossible to disentangle cause and effect.

Concern about the effects of alcohol on foetus the during pregnancy has also been expressed although, again, the amount of intake required to produce damage in the absence of confounding factors is debatable (Plant, 1985). A study of mortality in alcohol-dependent patients showed an overall death rate in excess of the expected value by a factor of 2.7 in men and 3.1 in women (Sherlock, 1982).

British mortality data indicate a very strong link between occupation and death from cirrhosis of the liver. These, however, do not show particular trends by social class, the highest risk group being publicans, closely followed by ship's personnel, barmen and barmaids, fishermen and hotel proprietors. Medical practitioners have three times the expected death rate from cirrhosis (OPCS, 1978).

A study of middle-aged men drawn from different parts of Britain found a progressive increase in drinking from social class I to V. Non-manual workers were the most likely to be light drinkers. These differences were apparent after controlling for town of residence. The data also indicated a strong relationship between smoking and drinking patterns, with moderate to heavy smoking being closely allied to moderate to heavy drinking (Cummins *et al.*, 1981). On the other hand, a study of patterns of referral to a clinic for alcohol abusers showed that the higher social classes were overrepresented in the clientele (Shaw and Thomas, 1977).

It is possible that figures which compare the reporting of the amount of alcohol consumed by manual and non-manual workers are biased by underreporting on the part of heavy drinkers (Popham, 1970). This may be especially significant in that heavy drinking may be less socially acceptable in middle-class groups, with the result that non-manual groups who do drink heavily would be more likely to underestimate their intake. More affluent individuals may also have more resources for concealing or buffering excessive intake of alcohol. It is possible that it is the social visibility of alcohol abuse which varies between classes rather than the extent.

Diet

Dietary imbalances due to the overconsumption of saturated fats, refined carbohydrates and salt, together with an underconsumption of unrefined foods such as fibre, have been linked to several medical conditions including coronary heart disease, obesity, diabetes, colon cancer and hypertension. The conclusions of the NACNE report were that the public should consume less animal fat, sugar and salt and increase its intake of fibre and polyunsaturated fats (NACNE, 1983).

Comparisons between countries have shown a positive relationship between the proportion of energy derived from saturated fats and mortality from coronary heart disease. Within-country data show a positive relationship between total plasma cholesterol and the incidence of coronary heart disease and there is some suggestion that a reduction in plasma cholesterol is associated with a reduced or even reversed progression of atherosclerotic lesions in femoral and coronary arteries (DHSS, 1984).

Salt intake has been linked to high blood pressure, although it is not clear why this should be the case. Cross-cultural studies show an association between average salt intake and average blood pressure in a population, but not within groups (WHO, 1983).

Burkitt (1980) has consistently maintained that the incidence of colon cancer could be cut dramatically by increasing the intake of dietary fibre. Fibre has also been said to influence blood concentration of cholesterol (Royal College of Physicians, 1980).

Obesity associated with excessive energy intake and low output is a risk factor for coronary heart disease, particularly in younger men, and being overweight is associated with increased risk of hypertension and diabetes (Royal College of Physicians, 1983).

Surprisingly little information is available about the food habits of individuals, outside the national surveys which, in any case, probably hide area and socioeconomic differences. Local surveys have found evidence for a poorer diet in low-income groups. Unable to buy expensive cuts of meat, people may compensate by purchasing poorer quality mince, sausages and meat pies, all of which are high in saturated fats (Cole Hamiton and Lang, 1986). A study in Manchester indicated that undernutrition was linked to low income (Lang, 1984). Indeed, it has been calculated that the cost of the diet recommended in the NACNE report is outside the income of poorer families altogether (Hunt, 1985).

A nationwide survey of 15–25-year-olds found intake of nutrients to be higher in higher social classes. For women, in particular, there was a decline in energy and nutrient intake from the highest to the lowest social classes (Bull and Barber, 1985). Moreover, in poorer areas outside urban centres, access to fresh fruit and vegetables may be limited both by availability and by cost (Hunt et al., 1987).

A sample of 6000 housewives in Britain showed that both younger and older women from semiskilled and unskilled occupational groups had diets high in butter, cheese and eggs, salt and confectionery, but low in fibre and low fat products (D'Arcy et al., 1986). There is an association between the consumption of sugar and sugar-containing products and low income (Ministry of Agriculture, Fisheries and Food, 1976). However, in general, it can be said that although diet and health may show some links at a population level, the evidence that there is an association at the individual level is almost entirely absent.

The Inadequacy of Behavioural Explanations

In relation to the four 'risk factors' it would seem that where they co-exist the absolute risk would be higher. However, due to the tendency for research to focus upon only one or two factors at a time it is impossible to know whether all four tend to cluster in the same people. It does seem that both the evidence that individual behaviours have a strong aetiological role and that they are differentially distributed according to social class remains equivocal.

The attempt to attribute higher sickness and mortality rates in the lower social classes and in certain geographical areas to behavioural factors effectively removes the social component from the aetiology of disease. Health and responsibility for health become individualized (Bartley, 1985) even though explanations for differences between social classes are usually at the group level.

There are fundamental flaws in the behavioural model of illness causation. There appears to be very little strong evidence that the patterning of the so-called 'risk behaviours' mirrors that of morbidity and mortality. Moreover, some of the behaviours in question are more likely to be markers or indicators of exposure to occupational, economic and environmental hazards, rather than the actual causes of illness.

The acceptance of a behavioural model has resulted in distortion and bias in the classification and even diagnosis of certain diseases. Moreover, disparities in standardized mortality ratios continue throughout life being most marked in the perinatal period but present at every age and for the vast majority of disease categories, even those to which individual behaviours have never been linked.

It seems evident that although some behaviours do play a part in the aetiology of some disorders, the weight of the individual component is quite unclear and, certainly, cannot account for differences between groups in relation to risk of disease. This will be illustrated by reference to three particular areas: perinatal mortality, coronary heart disease and lung cancer.

Perinatal mortality

The way in which a focus on individual behaviour may distract attention from more relevant factors in the social structure is well illustrated by class differences in perinatal mortality. Social class differences in mortality can be found at all ages but are most apparent in the period around birth. Perinatal mortality rates, that is, stillbirths and deaths in the first week of life, are almost two and a half times higher for babies born to social class V than to social class I parents (DHSS, 1980). This fairly constant difference remains against a background of dramatic improvements in perinatal mortality rates overall. Behavioural factors on the part of the mother which have been put forward as an explanation of social class differences in perinatal mortality include smoking during pregnancy (Simpson, 1957), poor diet (Rush, 1981), and late or no antenatal care (Hall et al., 1980). Women in social class V, for example, are somewhat more likely to first attend for antenatal care after the twentieth week of pregnancy (Brotherston et al., 1976). A variety of factors influence the seeking of medical care during pregnancy – including ease of access, the availability of childcare facilities, cost and the acceptability of services (Cartwright and Anderson, 1981). All of these may be more problematic for working-class women who have the least access to social and economic resources. However, the preventive and remedial value of routine antenatal care has been questioned (Hall et al., 1980), suggesting that late booking is an inadequate explanation for social class differences in perinatal mortality. A more plausible argument is that late antenatal attendence is an indicator or marker of poor social and living conditions and that these, not the implied fecklessness of social class V mothers-to-be, are the factors implicated in perinatal mortality rates. International 'league tables' for perinatal mortality are considered to be important and valid indicators of a country's health record (Office of Health Economics, 1978); it seems unlikely that antenatal care is the main reason for the difference between Third World and Western nations with respect to their perinatal mortality figures. On the other hand, there is some evidence that changes in the manner in which antenatal services are organized can influence both the acceptability of those services and perinatal outcome. Within a deprived area of Edinburgh with a perinatal mortality rate much above the national and Edinburgh level, a change from a system of city hospital to community-based antenatal care resulted in a marked decline in perinatal mortality (McKee, 1984). How far this was due to improved medical management or improved personal care is unclear, but recent intervention programmes suggest that social support during pregnancy can have beneficial effects on birth weight (Spencer, 1987).

Low birth weight is a major factor in perinatal mortality (Adelstein *et al.*, 1976) and accounts for much of the variation in mortality rates between the social classes (Office of Health Economics, 1978). Cigarette-smoking during pregnancy has been associated with birthweight decrements (Simpson, 1957). Women in manual social classes are about twice as likely to be smoking at term than middle-class women; more than 50% of women in social class V continue to smoke during pregnancy compared with less than a quarter of women in social class I. It is, therefore, inferred that smoking is a major cause of perinatal mortality and 'explains' social class variations. A recent study found that smoking was associated with a mean decrement of 215g in birth weight and this varied little across the social classes (Rush and Cassano, 1983). However, the authors found that only 37% of the association of birth weight with social class could be attributed to differences in smoking habits across class and, more importantly, that smoking was only associated with excess perinatal mortality among women in the lower, manual social classes. Moreover, smoking accounted for only a quarter of the social class difference in perinatal mortality. In other words, although smoking during pregnancy certainly affects birthweight this does not seem to be particularly harmful for the babies of middle-class smokers. Most of the excess perinatal mortality for lower social groups cannot be attributed to smoking. Smoking during pregnancy is not, *per se*, linked to perinatal mortality but must be mediated by other class-related variables, such as, poor diet, bad housing, lack of sleep and a minimum of social support.

Coronary heart disease

High on the list of diseases believed to have a largely behavioural aetiology is coronary heart disease (CHD). CHD is the most common cause of death in men (Townsend and Davidson, 1982) and its incidence and mortality rates vary by social class and geographical region (Shaper *et al.*, 1981; Barker and Osmond, 1987). The individual behaviours most often cited as increasing the risk of CHD are, as has been noted, diet (particularly dietary fats), cigarette-smoking, alcohol consumption and physical inactivity.

Bartley (1985) has drawn attention to some of the ways in which definitions of CHD have, over the years, become individualized. She suggested that this process grew out of an attempt to explain why, even with the development of a welfare state which was believed to be a great equalizer, inequalities in health remained. 'The idea of CHD as caused by obesity and sloth in the newly-affluent working classes fitted the requirements' (p. 290). There is, however, little evidence that differences in CHD mortality can be wholly attributed to differences in individual behaviour such as smoking, diet or exercise. The Whitehall study of civil servants, for example, showed that the lower the grade of employment the higher the rate of death from CHD, which was responsible for 43% of all deaths during the study period. However, differences in terms of 'risk factors', for example, smoking and plasma cholesterol levels, proved to be poor predictors of differences in mortality and could only account for about a third of the variation in relative risk between the highest and lowest Civil Service grades. Within categories of smokers there was a strong inverse relationship between mortality and employment grade for both CHD and lung cancer (Rose and Marmot, 1981). A differential effect for smoking in different groups has also been demonstrated by Haynes *et al.* (1980) who found that smoking was associated with CHD among male blue-collar workers but not among white-collar workers or women. Findings from the British Regional Heart Study (Shaper *et al.*, 1981) also indicate that behavioural factors cannot explain much of the social class and regional variation in CHD. Although alcohol intake and smoking rates were found to be related to blood pressure and cardiovascular disease, the data were correlational. There was a correlation within the 24 towns studied between the percentage of heavy smokers and drinkers, blood pressure and CHD mortality, but it was not demonstrated that those who smoked or drank the most were, in fact, those dying of CHD. Several studies have now shown that modest daily alcohol consumption has little or no detrimental health consequences and may even have a small preventive effect for fatal CHD (Hennekens *et al.*, 1978).

A prospective study in Sweden (Tibblin *et al.*, 1975) indicated that many so-called risk factors may be differentially related to fatal and non-fatal CHD. The authors suggest that their findings may indicate a non-specific influence of risk factors on different forms of heart disease or that the risk factor pattern '. . . merely mirrors a general liability to greater risk of disease' (p. 522).

The supposed link between dietary factors and CHD relates to the consumption of dietary lipids. These are thought to elevate serum cholesterol levels and cholesterol deposits on artery walls are postulated to be responsible for the atherosclerotic plaques and atherosclerosis which, in turn, 'cause' CHD. This chain of events, however, has been strongly disputed by Mitchell (1985). He argues, first that atherosclerosis is not synonymous with lipid deposition; secondly, that serum cholesterol levels are poor predictors of CHD and are, themselves, determined more by genetic than dietary factors, and thirdly, that dietary changes within populations have little influence on cholesterol levels and even less impact on rates of CHD.

Attempts to alter dietary practices and other behaviours provide useful supporting evidence for these criticisms as well as insights into the effects of behaviour and the interventions themselves on health outcomes. Overall, the data do not provide convincing support for the role of individual behaviour as an explanation of CHD. In relation to diet, experimental trials indicate that the introduction of low-cholesterol, low-saturated fat diets may result in some decrease in serum cholesterol levels among experimental groups, but that total mortality in control and experimental groups is almost identical (Dayton *et al.*, 1969; Turpeinen *et al.*, 1979). Any reductions in cardiovascular deaths are balanced by an increase in non-cardiovascular deaths (Mitchell, 1985). This pattern emerges from intervention trials which have attempted to control or change a variety of so-called risk factors through mass intervention.

The Multiple Risk Factor Intervention Trial (MRFIT) in America and the North Karelia project in Finland, mentioned in Chapter 5, are two such trials. In the American trial 'high risk' individuals were allocated to either an experimental group which was subject to multiple attempts to alter the 'risky' behaviours or to a control group which was not treated in this way (MRFIT Research Group, 1982). In the North Karelia project an entire community served as the experimental group for an ambitious project, which was developed out of concern for the very high rates of CHD in Finland (Vartiaine, et al.1986).

Although the prevalence of the risk behaviours in experimental groups or areas decreased, this also occurred in the control groups (Oliver, 1982) and must raise doubts about the effectiveness of mass interventions as a means of changing behaviour (Mitchell, 1985). More importantly, although the incidence of CHD declined, the trials indicate that there were few differences in overall mortality between experimental and control groups or areas: any decline in cardiovascular mortality is matched by an increase in deaths from other causes. In the USA, mortality from CHD has fallen by 25% (Harper, 1983) but this decline is apparent among all sections of the population. Similarly, Finland as a whole – not just North Karelia – has witnessed great reductions in cardiovascular mortality over the past 10 years and, as noted in Chapter 5, it has been suggested that it is improvements in the general standard of living and housing conditions in the past 10 years which are responsible for this decline in CHD rather than behavioural change *per se* (Rimpela, 1987). Similarly, Mitchell (1985) remains '. . . unconvinced that a poor black elderly woman living in Washington is likely to have changed her life style or been offered the advances in blood-pressure control and coronary care to the same extent as a young, affluent white man from Scarsdale' (p. 356).

Lung cancer

Although almost all causes of death show a clear social class gradient (DHSS, 1980), differences in individual behaviour are cited or implied as explanatory of class differences in incidence, for only some diseases. For example, lung cancer and many other diseases including emphysema, have been attributed almost wholly to cigarette smoking even though several studies have indicated that occupational exposure to, for example, coke-oven emissions (Doll *et al.* 1965) or uranium (Lundin, *et al.* 1971) are also major aetiological agents in lung cancer. It could even be suggested that the acceptance of an individualized behavioural model has itself resulted in behaviour alone being regarded as a principal variable for diagnostic purposes. Hammond and Selikoff (1975) in a study of lung cancer rates among asbestos workers have claimed that lung cancer rates are raised only among asbestos workers who smoke. A reanalysis of their data, however, indicated that although lung cancer rates among asbestos workers who smoked was about 10 times higher than among non-smoking asbestos workers, cancer mortality rates for both groups were almost identical (Sterling, 1978). Either smoking protected these workers against mesothelioma and other cancers or other factors are operating. Sterling suggests that an obvious interpretation is that physicians may be more inclined to diagnose lung cancer in someone who is a smoker than in someone who is not a smoker. He concludes that '. . . we do not find support for claims that smoking is the major hazard to workers' lungs' and suggests that smoking appears to have been used to divert attention away from the effects of occupational and environmental exposures' (p. 450).

Smoking is more common among some manual workers. For this reason it is often assumed that smoking is the main difference between manual and non-manual workers with respect to health. Yet, smoking is merely one of many differences between these groups. Manual workers are more likely to work in a dirty environments, to be exposed to air pollution, to live in poor housing, and to be on a low income to name but a few of the hazards they face. Indeed, Friedman *et al.* (1973) found that smokers are more likely to work in occupations which have a much higher exposure to industrial hazards-particularly fumes and dust than non-smokers. It is argued that any relationship between smoking and disease could mask a relationship between type of employment and disease, and that '. . . smoking in a statistical sense may be a major index for an individual exposed to occupational hazards in his employment' (Sterling, 1978, p. 448).

One possibility then is that smoking and other behaviours are, to a great extent, simply markers of other differences between the social classes. The use of tobacco and alcohol, for example, have been referred to as 'drugs of solace' (Cameron and Jones, 1985) which are a response to and a way of coping with stress and deprivation (Graham, 1986). Thus, although cigarette smoking may well play a role in the aetiology of some diseases, it also acts as an indicator of other, perhaps more important factors, such as hazardous work, bad housing, unemployment, low income, chronic fatigue and so on, either singly or, more likely, in combination. People in the lowest income groups are often burdened with multiple problems which impose continual strain upon their ability to cope. It has been suggested that rather than being primary causes of ill health, many so-called health-damaging behaviours are intervening variables and that observed associations between behaviour and mortality are largely fallacious (Blane, 1985). The risk of death for those on inadequate incomes has been found to be considerably higher than for those with more adequate incomes, even after standardizing for smoking, alcohol consumption, exercise and other behavioural factors (Slater *et al.*, 1985).

Social Class, Deprivation and Disadvantage

As has already been indicated analyses by social class are unsatisfactory for a variety of reasons and, in particular, they hide the very great differences within classes which are known to exist.

The introduction of the concept of deprivation has enabled the delineation of the more specific social circumstances associated with adverse health experiences. People who own their own home, for example, have lower mortality rates than those who live in privately-rented or local authority housing (DHSS, 1980). The combination of various indices of deprivation has been found to be particularly valuable. Holterman (1975), using eighteen indicators including housing type, employment status, financial assets and socioeconomic structure of the area, showed that the characteristics of deprivation were: poor housing, higher than average unemployment, low car ownership, more children in the age range 0–14 years and fewer elderly people than the average, more people from the New Commonwealth and more privately-rented accommodation than the mean for Great Britain.

These characteristics in various combinations have been associated with significant risk of health problems. Using simple epidemiology, Madeley (1978) found that post-neotnatal deaths tended to group together in certain parts of Nottingham, as did admissions to special care units because of failure to thrive, and non-accidental injuries. The associated areas were high on indicators of social deprivation.

Murphy *et al.* (1982) found a close association between sudden infant death and deprived families from poor areas, especially where the mother was young and of high parity. The male suicide rate by means other than domestic gas in the period 1955–80 showed a strong positive correlation with unemployment (Kreitman and Platt, 1984). The suicides did not necessarily occur among the unemployed, but rather appeared to indicate general distress and that loosening of social cohesion in a community suggested by Durkheim (1897).

Both males and females from deprived areas exhibit a pattern of morbidity more appropriate to older age groups (Boddy, 1983). An analysis carried out in Edinburgh and Glasgow by Carstairs (1981), using seven Census variables; overcrowding (more than two people to a room), lack of amenities, low social class, unemployment, economic activity, car ownership and number of rooms, showed a moderate to strong correlation between the deprivation index and standardized mortality rates in the areas, the rate of discharges from hospital, bed-days, mental hospital admissions and the percentage of live birth weights below 5.5 pounds. Infectious diseases, respiratory infections and accidents were strongly associated with the indices of deprivation, but associations were not significant for perinatal or infant mortality.

Different forms of family life may also play a role in vulnerability to health problems. Deprived areas are characterized by an excess number of single-parent families. Wadsworth *et al.* (1983) have shown that children in single-parent families and those with step-parents are more likely to suffer accidental injury in the first 5 years of life. Blaxter and Paterson (1982) found that in their sample of families from low-income areas 51% of male children and 43% of female children under 9 years of age were suffering from one or more chronic conditions such as otitis media, squint, deafness, eczema enuresis and urinary infections. Children from disadvantaged families are three times more likely to come into contact with mental health personnel, one in three never attend a child health clinic and only one-third of the rest attend regularly. They are less likely to be protected against polio and diphtheria, have more absences from school through illness, have more accidents and are four times more likely to suffer from hearing loss (Wedge and Prosser, 1973). Their hospitalization rates are higher and number of bed-days greater than for non-deprived children (Egbuonal and Starfield, 1982).

These relative disparities between groups of families and the deficit in child health in the most deprived groups may well persist through into adult life for a significant proportion (Butler and Alderman, 1969; Brotherston, 1976; Blaxter, 1981). The greater the number of indications of deprivation, the more acute and intransigent are the health problems (Davie *et al.*, 1972; Wedge and Prosser, 1973; Court Report, 1976).

Illsley and Mullen (1985) have reviewed the subcategories which can be described as deprived and/or disadvantaged. These comprise the low paid, the unemployed, one-parent families, the elderly, ethnic minorities, the chronically ill and the mentally and physically handicapped. However, a survey by Townsend (1979) found that 22% of households living in poverty did not belong to any of these groups and it is clear that not all members of such groups will be deprived. The association of ill health with these categories is related to the position of their members in the social structure, their educational background, the opportunities available and access to resources and power.

General susceptibility

Of all the explanations given for the links between deprivation/disadvantage and ill health the one which best fits the empirical data and the little available theory is that of general susceptibility. Chapter 1 has drawn attention to the focus of epidemiology on disease-specific factors. Cassell (1976) has argued that a disease-a specific orientation has caused investigators to miss the importance of the complex of diseases as a whole. The fact that a very wide range of diseases and disorders is associated with a particular group of people has received insufficient attention from both a medical and a political perspective. It has been pointed out that diseases such as lung cancer, arthritis, diabetes, heart disease, bronchitis and so on are seen to be inherent in individuals regardless of the fact that individuals come and go from the population where these diseases are most likely to occur (Syme, 1986). Deprivation and disadvantage have been associated for centuries with excess mortality and morbidity in spite of huge changes in behaviour, the gene pool, marriage patterns, social mobility, political and economic cycles, and medical provision. The important question thus becomes what do the disadvantaged and the deprived have in common now, which is similar, in essence, to what they have had in common, historically and geographically?

The poor have, of course, always been more likely to inhabit a physical environment, at work and at home which is much more unpleasant than that of their more affluent compatriots. This is illustrated by the Edinburgh tenements, an early version of high rise, in the seventeenth, eighteenth and nineteenth centuries, when the rich lived on the top floors and threw their garbage and excrement into the streets below, sometimes on to the very heads of the poor, who lived on the lowest levels. Here they were not only deprived of light and air, but were also subject to the unpleasantness piling up in front of their doors – a situation not only factual but poignantly symbolic. Even in rural areas, the hovels and cottages of the workers were damp, crowded and unhygienic. The towns were also crowded with large numbers of homeless who were forced to sleep in the noisome streets. From the time of the Industrial Revolution the work of the low-paid was hard, long, virtually without holidays and likely to lead to an early death for many from accidents in mills, mines and factories and from the inhalation of noxious substances, as well as from the long hours of labour combined with inadequate nutrition.

The rise of the public health movement and various Acts of Parliament did much to alleviate the worst aspects of housing and the work place. The effect of public health measures on mortality and morbidity has been well documented by McKeown (1976). Nevertheless, those whose incomes are low are still more likely to live in poor housing which may be damp, cold or noisy, or all three and to have few resources to remedy the situation. If they are in work at all, they are more likely to have jobs which expose them to some health hazard.

Housing

From the mid-nineteenth century to the 1950s the connection between poor housing and health was scarcely in doubt. Indeed, an analysis of housing conditions formed a regular part of the annual report of most medical officers of health. The earliest local authority housing was designed with health in mind, providing access to open spaces for recreation, with a sunny aspect and adequate rooms for the size of family. A description of the design of some working-class cottages makes the point very well:

> Mr Parker (the architect) has always before his mind the following facts: A tuberculosis germ will live for two years out of the direct rays of the sun and not more than ten minutes in the sun. A typhoid germ has the same life out of the sun and two minutes in the sun. He regards a through living-room – i.e. one with a window at each end – as indispensable. . . . (Weaver, 1926)

The relationship of tuberculosis to housing conditions led to vigorous campaigns for the irradication of overcrowding and the provision of adequate heat and light.

With the decline of TB as a significant public health problem, interest in housing as an aetiological factor in disease diminished dramatically and, in Britain, people from slum clearances were hustled into mass housing projects, hastily, carelessly and cheaply built without consideration for the physical or mental health of the inhabitants. Housing tenure has consistently been associated with morbidity and mortality (DHSS, 1980).

One explanation for the decline in concern with housing conditions may be that the National Health Service with its curative and hospital orientation engendered disinterest in, and a lack of resources for, prevention. Another reason may be that the decrease in infectious disease associated with housing means that any problems which might be related to living conditions are not of a type likely to spread to the houses of the middle and upper classes.

Currently, interest in the links between housing and health is reviving but it is fascinating to observe the reluctance to consider such links, on the grounds that a direct link betwen housing *per se* and health problems has not been conclusively demonstrated, (e.g. Pike, 1982). Considering the speed with which other much more tenuous factors quickly become part of the mythology of the aetiology of disease, for example, the consumption of saturated fats, this demand for 'proof' begins to look tendentious.

Some of the difficulties associated with establishing causal links between housing and ill health stem from the focus on cases of disease referred to earlier. If one defines 'health' as does WHO (1948) then bad housing can clearly be established as affecting physical mental and social well-being.

A longitudinal study of people who had been rehoused from slum dwellings showed improved health after 3 years as compared with a control group (Wilner *et al.*, 1982). The relationship between overcrowding and respiratory disease is well established (McMillan, 1957; Brennan and Little, 1979; B. Stephens *et al.*, 1985). Chest conditions, including asthma, rhinitis and alveolitis have been fairly conclusively related to the presence of fungal spores in damp housing (Hosen, 1978; Maunsel, 1954; Strachan and Elton, 1986). Martin (*et al.*, 1987), using a double blind design, established that the prevalence of reported symptoms such as cough, wheeze, diarrhoea, vomiting, fatigue, headaches, aches and pains, was significantly greater for children in damp housing as compared to those in dry. They were able to rule out smoking, income, reporting bias and types of heating as contributory factors to the findings. Damp and cold houses, conditions which are exacerbated by inability to afford sufficient heating, foster fungal contamination, the extent of which, in its effects on health, is largely unknown, but probably serious. In addition, damp encourages the proliferation of house mites which give rise to allergies, and bacteria which may cause infections (Lacey *et al.*, 1972).

Approximately 30% of local authority housing in the North of England and Scotland suffers some degree of damp, causing internal pollution. There is little doubt that many of the inhabitants of these houses also belong to deprived and disadvantaged groups.

Working conditions

A large number of manual occupations are known directly to affect health (Pochin, 1973), although the incidence of industrial disease is hard to assess since there is a reluctance to specify that medical conditions are work-related because of the fear of claims for compensation. Factory workers are exposed to chemicals, noise and dust, continuing contact with which can lead to a variety of disorders (Hunter, 1975). Assembly-line work has been linked to stress-related symptoms, such as facial tics, fatigue and irritability (Timio et al., 1979). Jobs with little or no decision latitude, where pace and type of movements are externally controlled and job satisfaction is virtually nil, have been associated with increased risk of coronary heart disease (Karasek et al., 1981). The effect of pollution in the workplace on respiratory diseases has tended to take second place to the effects of smoking, but both Sterling (1978) and Cockcroft (1982) have produced data to show that lung cancer and emphysema are related to working conditions even when smoking is controlled for.

Blane (1985) has suggested that there is evidence that deaths from occupational exposure to dangerous conditions are under recorded. Certainly, Cochrane and Moore (1981) succeeded in demonstrating that deaths from pneumoconiosis were under reported by approximately 60%. Not only are the workers exposed to hazardous substances, but they may take contaminants home on their clothing and skin. It has been calculated that about 20% of the social class variation in cancer mortality arises directly from hazards at work (Fox and Adelstein, 1978) and some writers believe that up to 40% of deaths from cancer will soon be attributable to the work environment (Davies, 1982).

Unemployment

The handicapped, the low-paid, older people and unskilled workers are more likely to become unemployed. The OPCS longitudinal study shows that mortality is increased in men who are seeking work and that this cannot be accounted for by previous illness or by social class (Moser et al., 1984). Using data from the General Household Surveys of 1981 and 1982, Arber (1987) showed that low social class and non-employment are independently associated with ill health, although there is considerable overlap. She concluded that social class affects the health of the jobless to an even greater extent than it does those in employment. The few longitudinal studies which have followed workers through from employment to unemployment do suggest physiological changes such as increased levels of circulating hormones, cholesterol, noradrenalin and creatinine. In addition, elevated blood pressure, colds, ulcers and arthritis were observed more frequently after unemployment (Kasl et al., 1975; Cobb and Kasl, 1977). Some studies have found higher rates of self-reported illnesses in the unemployed, and higher frequencies of chest complaints and heart disease, depression and use of tranquillizers (Fagin and Little, 1981; Cook et al., 1982).

A study of unemployment among bricklayers showed that just as hospital admission increased the risk of unemployment, so unemployment increased the risk of hospital admission. This investigation did not support the contention that only men with more ill health were more likely to become unemployed (Lajer, 1982).

The experience of unemployment does give rise to measurable stress effects particularly in relation to the sympathetic nervous system. The effects may result in a variety of physical, emotional and behavioural changes including vulnerability to illness, impairment of performance and 'learned helplessness' which ensues upon attempting to get work and constantly failing (Baum et al., 1986).

Environmental conditions

People with low levels of disposable income, especially those belonging to deprived groups, have diminished opportunity to choose where they will live and inhabit disproportionately the disadvantaged areas of the inner cities or housing estates on the periphery of towns. Each of these locations has its own disadvantages. Inner-city areas will be noisy, dirty and polluted. Peripheral estates usually lack amenities for shopping and recreation. Food prices tend to be higher. Both locations suffer, often, from vandalism, litter and a depressing aspect. Safe playing areas for children are limited and it is well established that children of socially deprived parents are at greater risk of both domestic and road accidents (Brown and Davidson, 1978; Backett, 1975). There is a link between air pollution and adult respiratory disease (Colley et al., 1973) and between local industrial pollution and elevated lung cancer rates (Gardner et al., 1982).

Naturally, these adverse life circumstances are not isolated the one from the other. For example, families are twice as likely to live in overcrowded conditions when the father is unemployed (Brennan and Lancashire, 1978). Communities with poor housing tend to contain more unemployed people and to be located in a physical environment which is both hazardous and aesthetically unpleasant.

Deprived individuals are exposed to several risk factors simultaneously, often for long periods of time, any one of which may make them more vulnerable to one or more of the others. Colley and Reid (1970) found that the effect of air pollution on childhood respiratory disease was apparent only for social classes IV and V. Brennan and Lancashire (1978) established a significant and positive relationship between mortality in children aged 0–4 years, low socioeconomic status, high-density housing, poor amenities and the unemployment rate.

An analysis of mortality rates in three neighbouring towns in Lancashire indicated that much of the variance in mortality between the towns was accounted for by ischaemic heart disease, chronic bronchitis, stroke or bronchopneumonia (Barker and Osmond, 1987). Lung cancer rates in these towns were at the national average or below. The authors concluded that 'differences in mortality between the three towns were almost entirely due to socioeconomic differences and that past differences in maternal health and physique and in the postnatal environment, particularly infant feeding, housing and overcrowding, may be determinants of current differences in adult mortality' (p. 752).

In addition to the stress emanating from the physical environment, low-income families are less able to buffer the strains of everyday life because of their inability to afford adequate nutrition, heating in winter and an appropriate level of comfort. It has been suggested that this inability of the less affluent to protect themselves from cold and damp, e.g. by adequate housing, heating and food, may modify physiological or biochemical parameters and that this may account for the excess levels of ischaemic heart disease in cold and damp areas (West and Lowe, 1976).

Regardless of specific disease outcomes, it should be apparent that living with social and economic disadvantage imposes daily strains often upon people who lack adequate resources of education, access to powerful groups, and social support.

The occurrence of 'life-events' has been associated with increased risk of illness by associating 'life-change scores' to illness risk (Holmes and Masuda, 1974; Theorell *et al.*, 1975). This model has been criticized on a number of grounds: e.g. that positive associations have most often been found by retrospective accounts, that associations have generally accounted for less than 10% of the variance and that the model ignores individual differences in coping and perception of the significance of the event (Andrews and Tennant, 1978). However, the work on life-events does draw attention to the concept of 'general susceptibility' to illness as opposed to a disease-specific model. Numerous studies have shown that mortality and morbidity rates exhibit patterning, not only in relation to social class, but also for marital status, occupational rank, religious affiliation, education and so on (Berkson, 1962; Keehn, 1974; Fuchs, 1974).

A general susceptibility theory of illness suggests that some combination of life circumstances and experiences either precipitates or predisposes to illness in some sections of the population. This theory has its roots in the work of Selye (1950), who postulated that human beings are subject to a 'general adaptation syndrome' which arises as a consequence of strains imposed upon the person's ability to adapt both physically and mentally to those strains and to cope with them. Events which tax the person's ability to cope give rise to detectable physiological and biochemical changes. Where these changes are prolonged the immunological system becomes less viable. There is, indeed, a great deal of evidence to support this contention. Catecholamine and corticosteroid output increases under stress (Frankenhaeuser, 1975; Rose, 1980; Dimsdale and Moss, 1980) and both of these can impair immunological functioning (Gruchow, 1979; Bach *et al.*, 1975; Strom and Carpenter, 1980).

There is now a considerable body of research which demonstrates how social conditions and their sequelae can affect the body's defence system, by interfering with immunocompetence (for an excellent review, see Jemmott and Locke, 1984). The poorer sections of the population inhabit a social and physical environment which imposes daily strains in a constant and prolonged manner. Their lives are characterized by problems of money, uncomfortable housing, noise and litter, worries about work, family and health, encounters with bureaucracy, inadequate clothing and food and this, often, without the prospect of a break, not even for a weekend, never mind a fortnight in the Camargue. Such circumstances are not so much composed of discrete life events, rather, life is one long series of interacting events and myriad frustrations which tax the ability to cope to the maximum and beyond. It is not so surprising that people may require 'drugs of solace' (Cameron and Jones, 1985) to help them through the day.

The deprived and disadvantaged live in an environment which is not only physically unhealthy, but which contains an excessive amount of social and psychological strain. The disadvantaged are subjected to all the exigencies of the human condition, plus those extra contingencies which tend to arise for people who lack adequate funds, education, privilege and social power. Without the buffers provided by these latter resources individuals in deprived areas must cope with a great many long-and short-term problems.

As has been argued, the evidence for the contribution of behavioural factors to illness is rather sparse and, in some cases, suspect. Certainly, the impact of behaviour on health is likely to be far less than that which ensues upon living under conditions of social deprivation. Certainly 'drugs of solace' may make a contribution to the whole complex of factors leading to breakdowns in health, especially in vulnerable groups. Such groups are likely to be more susceptible than others to a wide variety of specific toxins and disease agents including viruses and air pollutants. Gross poverty, grinding labour and the filthy hovels of the past may no longer exist, but certainly social, educational, environmental and psychological impoverishment is not uncommon, providing a modern version of the Marxist concept of 'immiseration'. Britain has been an inequitable society for centuries. That political, economic and social inequalities should manifest themselves in health differences should surprise no one. What is surprising is that such inequities should be attributed to differences in behaviour, when evidence for this view is grossly inadequate compared to the wealth of data which links them to social conditions. As Illsley and Mullen (1985) have pointed out, 'Low pay may be a salient characteristic of an individual but the existence of a large low-paid (and, it should be added, unemployed) population is a characteristic of society itself' (p. 98).

The health of deprived populations is unlikely to improve until such time as fundamental changes are made in the social structure. The likelihood of this emanating from the top must be regarded as infinitesimal. Other initiatives, however, such as those described in Chapter 8, may stand some chance of chipping away at existing inequalities through the efforts of people in deprived communities themselves.

CHAPTER 7

A Public Health Approach to Mental Well-Being

The evidence that psychological distress and mental illness are associated with adverse social conditions is now extensive, although establishing causal links between social factors and poor mental health is, as ever, problematic. However, many of the factors associated with psychological difficulties are not very different from those which have been linked with physical morbidity and mortality (see Chapter 6). The present chapter reviews some of the evidence with respect to mental health and suggests how psychological well-being might be promoted at the individual, the group and, particularly, the population level. Many of the salient issues are more fully discussed in the previous and the following chapters. The aim of this chapter, therefore, is to apply the data relating to social and health inequalities to the field of mental health and to suggest how public health principles might be developed.

Concepts and definitions of mental health are numerous: none, however, is wholly satisfactory since they tend to describe *ill* health rather than *well*-being and cover a range of heterogeneous phenomena. Almost inevitably, mental well-being is defined simply as the absence of 'illness'. It often seems that academic debate is more concerned with issues of diagnosis and whether different categories of psychological disturbance are manifestations of disease, illness or distress, rather than with issues of prevention and health promotion. In other words, as in the field of physical health, a medical model predominates.

The main focus of this chapter will be on depression and anxiety, whether or not these problems have come to the attention of the medical profession, rather than on serious, but relatively rare, psychotic illnesses which invariably require and result in medical treatment.

The Prevalence of Mental Ill Health

Differences in rates of mental disturbance reported in various studies are often simply a reflection of the fact that any estimate of the prevalence of mental ill health is dependent on sampling, definition and measurement. Psychiatric registers based on in-patient and out-patient consultations grossly underestimate the prevalence of psychological ill health in the community and are, therefore, inadequate and misleading indicators.

A striking feature of psychiatric surveys of random samples of the general population is the extent to which psychological distress is widespread in the population. General population surveys in Britain which have used standardized interview techniques and diagnostic criteria indicate that between 14% and 17% of the population is, at any one time, seriously or clinically depressed (Brown and Harris, 1978; Bebbington et al., 1981). Studies in Australia report prevalence rates of between 21% and 24% (Henderson et al., 1978; Tennant and Andrews, 1978). Thus, a considerable proportion of the population report not only persistent feelings of depression (such as feeling low, crying and unhappiness) but also difficulties such as sleep problems, loss of appetite, lethargy and feelings of hopelessness. If less severe forms of emotional distress are included, approximately a third of the population might be affected (Brown et al., 1975; Hunt et al., 1986). Few of these problems receive 'treatment' and, indeed, the factors which appear to increase the likelihood of mental health problems may also inhibit the same people from seeking help (Brown and Harris, 1978).

Rates of depression and/or anxiety for women are approximately twice those for men and this pattern remains constant whether the sample comprises depressed patients treated by a psychiatrist (Wing and Hailey, 1972) or cases identified in random community surveys (Warheit et al., 1973; Bebbington et al., 1981). Women with young children, particularly those who do not have paid employment outside the home, have especially high rates of depression. While Brown and Harris found that working-class women had considerably higher rates of distress than middle-class women, a psychiatric survey carried out in the same area (Camberwell, London) found a slight trend in that direction, but the association between social class and psychiatric disorder was not significant (Bebbington et al., 1981). The same methods were used in both surveys, to assess psychiatric disturbance and to measure social class. However, Brown's study only looked at women, whereas Bebbington's included men. Whereas Brown generally classified women's social class by husband's occupation the Bebbington study used women's own or most recent occupation. This has the result of putting more women into the non-manual categories. Differences in sampling may also account for the apparent discrepancy in the findings of the two studies.

An association between low social class and poor mental health has been demonstrated by a large number of studies which tap varying degrees of psychological disturbance (see Dohrenwend and Dohrenwend, 1969, for a review of early studies; for more recent studies see Comstock and Hesling, 1976, and Hunt et al., 1986). Although it has been argued that psychiatric hospital admissions are an inadequate index of mental ill health, social class differences are also evident in studies of psychiatric consultation rates. For example, a comparison of admission rates from different parts of the catchment area of a mental hospital found that the admission rate from the two most deprived electoral wards was six times that of the more affluent areas (Kangesu, 1984). Similarly, children from disadvantaged families are three times more likely to come into contact with mental health personnel (Wedge and Prosser, 1973). Such children tend to have a greater than expected number of psychosocial disorders, psychoses, personality disorders, behavioural and psychological problems and learning disabilities (Starfield *et al.*, 1980).

Some of the reasons why there may be a preponderance of mental ill health in lower social class groups are discussed below. However, the view that these associations are merely an artefact of 'downward social mobility' (i.e. that the mentally ill and psychologically disturbed simply move into low-status occupations and poor conditions as a result of their mental state) is probably only relevant with respect to chronic conditions like schizophrenia (Goldberg and Morrison, 1963) and, even here, findings that people with diagnosed psychotic illnesses move down the social scale are beset by methodological difficulty (Blane, 1985). Moreover, such arguments cannot explain why some ethnic groups have higher rates of mental illness than Caucasians born in Britain (Giggs, 1986).

Social Factors and Mental Health

Psychological disturbance in an individual may develop quite unexpectedly with no apparent antecedents. Although schizophrenic-type disorders – characterizd by halluci- nations, delusions and paranoia – often have a familial or genetic component, it is also the case that emotionally charged life-events may trigger the first episode of the illness (Brown and Birley, 1968). Moreover, aspects of social and family life may influence recovery and relapse rates (Vaughn and Leff, 1976). The role of life-events, however, has been most strongly demonstrated with respect to depressive-type disturbances. Although it might seem intuitively obvious that psychological distress is a reaction to an unpleasant event or set of circumstances, this is at variance with a medical model which defines mental disturbance as a manifestation of individual pathology or disease.

Threatening or unpleasant life-events in the recent past have been shown to play a crucial role in the development of depression. Differential exposure to life-events also appears to explain, in part, gender and social class differences in the experience of depression, the highest rates being found among working-class women (Brown *et al.*, 1975; Parry, 1986). These studies assessed the presence or absence of 'clinical' depression using a standardized psychiatric interview (the Present State Examination). Information about recent reported 'symptoms' was used in conjunction with diagnostic criteria to classify the sample as 'case depression', 'borderline depression' or 'normal'. It was intended that these classifications should approximate those used by psychiatrists and that those defined as cases should resemble, clinically, the people whom a psychiatrist would expect to treat on an in-patient or out-patient basis (Brown and Harris, 1978).

Social class differences were marked in Brown and Harris' large survey: whereas 23% of working-class women were found to be depressed in the 3 month period before interview, the same was true for only 6% of the middle-class women in the sample. This social class difference, however, was only apparent for women with children, suggesting that the experience of motherhood for many working-class women may be particularly stressful because of their circumstances. Brown and Harris found that working-class women had experienced a greater number of stressful life-events compared with middle-class women in relation to housing, their partner's job, finance or marriage. A recent study using the same methodology has confirmed the social class differences in life-event experience and relationship to the development of depression (Parry, 1986).

There is now a voluminous literature on life-events and their effect on mental health. Early studies suggested that the more life-events an individual experienced in a defined time period, the greater the likelihood of a depressive breakdown (e.g. Holmes and Rahe, 1967). The methodology employed in such studies assumed that particular events were of equivalent stress for individuals regardless of the desirability or undesirability of the event for that individual. Recent studies using more sophisticated measures, however, indicate that it is the *context* in which a particular event occurs which determines its likely stressfulness for an individual (Brown and Harris, 1978; Costello, 1982). The meaning of events is considered to be the more important aetiological consideration and that meaning itself is socially constructed (Brown, 1974). Thus the 'same' event, for example, the birth of a baby, means very different things depending on the circumstances in which it takes place.

Some groups appear to have a higher life-event rate than others; that is, they are more likely in a defined period to have experienced an event considered, because of it's context, to be stressful. Thus, working-class women have been found to have an especially high life-event rate and, moreover, appears to be particularly vulnerable to the negative effects of life events (Brown and Harris, 1978), in that they are more likely than middle-class women to break down after a crisis event.

It has to be remembered that life-events are often the end result or focus of long-term difficulties rather than discrete occurrences. For example, a family without anyone in paid employment experiencing extreme financial hardship may get increasingly into debt, be unable to pay their rent or mortgage and be evicted from their home. Although life-events are strongly implicated in the development of depression they do not, on their own, provide a full explanation or description of the complexity of the relationship between social factors and mental distress.

The greater vulnerability of working-class women appears to be due, in part, to the sometimes poor relationship with their partner at the time that they have young children, the number of children in the household and the lack of paid employment outside the home (Brown et al., 1975). Although Brown has argued that these factors mediate the effects of life-events, other studies have suggested that they are, in fact, causes or antecedents of depression in their own right (Tennant and Bebbington, 1978; Martin et al., 1982).

The role of social support in mental health has received considerable attention. Several studies have shown that lack of social support is associated with depression (Cobb, 1976; Henderson et al., 1978). The quality of supportive or affectual ties is seen as more important than the presence and number of social networks and contacts (Dean and Lin, 1977; Thoits, 1982). Brown's studies placed particular emphasis on the quality of relationships with a spouse or sexual partner as a factor which can protect an individual against the negative effects of stressful life-events, although it is clear that close or confiding ties with other people can also prevent or reduce the chance of becoming depressed at times of crisis (Miller and Ingham, 1976). Depression can also affect the quality of relationships and poor social support may sometimes be a consequence rather than an antecedent of mental distress (Mitchell and Moos, 1984).

Lack of, or inadequate, social support is obviously just one of a number of factors which explain why working-class women with children appear to be especially vulnerable to mental ill health. Brown and Harris found that, at the point in their lives when they are bringing up young children, working-class women appear to be less likely than middle-class women to have a close relationship with their husband. They attribute this to 'long-term cultural influences' concerning the division of labour and patterns of communication within working-class families. An alternative explanation which is merely alluded to is that working class women with young children are usually having to cope with many household and financial problems and that this may dominate to the extent that there is little time or energy to devote to the marriage. Intimacy appears to improve among working-class couples once they are no longer having to care for young children. Bebbington *et al.* (1981), however, have suggested that the high rates of depression among women with children may be due to their exclusion from the paid workforce; some of the effects of unemployment on mental health are discussed below.

A more general explanation is that many women caring for young children are isolated from others who are in a similar situation and often they receive little support from families and friends, in what can itself be a very stressful and demanding occupation (Richman, 1976). The particular vulnerability of some working-class mothers may also relate to more segregated gender roles, fewer opportunities to make contact with their families and friends because of transport problems and the generally greater adversity they may face because of poor housing, unemployment and poverty.

Unemployment and its sequelae are increasingly being associated with poor mental health in much the same way that they have been linked with physical morbidity and mortality. Indeed, analysis of unemployment and mortality rates in the OPCS longitudinal survey found that suicide was among the main causes of an increased mortality rate among the unemployed (Moser *et al.*, 1984). Other studies have also linked unemployment with both attempted and successful suicide (Platt, 1987).

A study which examined the mental health of employed and unemployed school-leavers found that the unemployed had higher levels of depression and anxiety than the employed even though the two groups were no different with respect to mental health when they left school. Those who had found employment but were subsequently made redundant deteriorated psychologically, while those who eventually found paid work improved (Banks and Jackson, 1982). This study provides fairly conclusive evidence for the causal effects of unemployment on mental health. Most studies have been mainly concerned with the effects of unemployment on men. A recent study of women with children did not find a striking effect for paid employment on their mental well-being (Parry, 1986). It is suggested that the benefits of employment outside the home are only apparent where social, financial and psychological needs are not met within the domestic role (Warr and Parry, 1982).

Warr (1984) identifies six principal benefits of paid employment to individuals and how loss or absence of these might affect their mental health. These are: money, raised activity levels, variety, temporal structure, social contacts and personal identity. The transition to unemployment, he argues, requires the unemployed person to adopt a new role which is both threatening and unpleasant. Hartley (1980) found that the unemployed tend to have lower self-esteem than the employed. Other studies have, similarly, shown that the unemployed have significantly reduced positive affect and feelings of pleasure, higher scores on measures of depression indicating a risk of psychiatric illness and lower life satisfaction (Banks and Jackson, 1982; Warr and Payne, 1982). The duration of unemployment is significantly associated with both depression and life satisfaction (Hepworth, 1980). Financial strain and problems – an obvious consequence of unemployment – are strongly associated with psychological distress (Warr, 1984) and were found to be a major factor associated with the development of depression in pregnancy (Martin et al., 1982).

A number of studies have shown that sub-standard or inappropriate housing is related to poor mental health and psychiatric illness. The rapid expansion of the public housing sector in the post-war years led to a great increase not only in inadequate housing but also to the placing of families with young children in blocks of flats with few facilities, either for the children or their mothers. Although slum clearance was and still is desperately needed, the mass movement into new, insensitively planned housing estates often resulted in the disruption of existing communities and the dislo-cation of families. A study of one of the new large housing estates in the 1950s found higher rates of 'neurosis' and psychiatric hospital admission among adults living in the flats compared with those living in more traditional houses on the same estate (Martin et al., 1957). The increased illness rates were thought to be due more to specific types of housing (flats as opposed to more traditional houses) than to stress associated with the move to the estate. Similarly, Fanning (1967) also found links between living in high-rise flats and mental distress, defined as psychiatric consultations. While a recent study of council house dwellers in Newcastle found that high-rise flats were associated with raised levels of distress the main effect on mental health was the area of residence (Byrne et al., 1986). Thus, those living in the worst neighbourhoods – for example, 'difficult-to-let' areas – had the poorest psychological health. Inevitably, housing conditions, housing type and area of residence are inter-related; a study of the health effects of living in one of the less desirable housing schemes in Edinburgh, found that mental distress was common among the tenants as a whole and was particularly high for those living in damp and mouldy houses. Children living in the damp houses also appeared to suffer more from problems such as 'nerves' than children living in the dry dwellings (Martin et al., 1987). In terms of severe psychological and psychiatric disturb-ance, housing problems have been found to be one of the main factors explaining relapse or poor recovery (Goldberg and Huxley, 1982).

The following sections examine the public health implications of the evidence that mental distress is related to social factors and outlines some of the ways in which mental health can be promoted at a population level.

Public Health Implications

While feelings of depression, anxiety and distress are experienced at an individual level, the factors largely associated with mental ill health are not individual but social. Poor housing conditions, unemployment, financial problems, isolation and lack of supportive agencies and networks are all implicated in mental health such that whole communities, because of their social structure, are vulnerable. Most people experiencing psychological distress do not consult their GP and, even if they do, problems are inevitably perceived and dealt with as located within that individual rather than being seen as a reflection of social 'disease'. Indeed, the most common response by many GPs and psychiatrists is the mass prescription of tranquillizers. This can usually only be a palliative measure and has itself resulted in a major health problem in terms of long-term dependency on these drugs and the experience of side-effects. The consumption of other potentially harmful products, such as tobacco and alcohol, is a further reflection of the conditions in which many people live and work, conditions which offer few choices or opportunities for change and over which people have little control (Cameron and Jones, 1985).

Colin Murray Parkes (1979) suggests, because most of the causal factors leading to or precipitating mental ill health are social circumstances which impinge on vulnerable sections of the community, '. . . it is therefore reasonable to suppose that the increased focusing of psychiatric resources in the community will begin to make it possible for psychiatrists to work with other community agents to develop preventive intervention programmes' (p. 50). Although many life-events cannot be prevented, others and their potentially negative effects can be predicted and intervention *before* a crisis actually occurs is sometimes possible. For example, studies indicate that 'anticipatory guidance' before a known event which is likely to be stressful can significantly reduce psychosocial or psychophysical problems (Carpenter *et al.*, 1968). Similarly, support and counseling after bereavement has been shown to reduce negative outcomes. In an experimental study, widows considered to be at high risk for psychological problems were divided into two groups, an experimental group receiving weekly counselling after their bereavement, and a control group who received no counselling. Compared with the controls, those receiving counselling made fewer visits to their doctor, had a lower consumption of alcohol, tobacco and tranquillizers and had fewer psychological symptoms (Raphael, 1977).

Although desirable, crisis intervention and post-event support do require the identification of those individuals most 'at risk'. How this could be achieved on anything other than a fairly small and localized scale is problematic. Moreover, by focusing on only specific events, the individualizing of stress-related problems may be perpetuated.

Mental Health Initiatives

An alternative strategy is to develop services which are locally based and, therefore, accessible to whole communities and to which people can refer themselves. An understanding of local events and problems could facilitate opportunities for professionals and lay workers to make themselves available when necessary. Some examples are given here of a few local initiatives, within a medical or quasi-medical setting, which attempt to provide community-based care which goes beyond, and may prevent, the need for formal psychiatric treatment.

In Tameside (Manchester) a comprehensive, community-based mental health centre has been established (Wooff *et al.*, 1983). The centre is managed communally by its staff and no one is designated as being in overall charge. The team includes social workers, psychiatrists, a psychologist, day-centre therapists, art therapists and a nursery nurse. Initial referrals are dealt with by either the social workers, psychiatrists or the psychologist and it is not assumed that all clients must see the doctor. The centre operates on an 'open-door' policy and hopes to divert people with emotional problems away from formal psychiatric services. Because of its psychosocial rather than medical orientation, the centre aims to move towards a greater preventive role. However, its identification as a psychiatric service may make this difficult.

The Mental Health Advice Centre in Lewisham (London) is staffed by professionals from a variety of backgrounds including psychiatry, clinical psychology, psychotherapy and social work, who are backed up by volunteers (Bouras and Brough, 1982). Again, clients may self-refer without an appointment. They will be seen by whichever professional is on duty and, later, a key worker will be selected to maintain contact with the client. Most of the clients who come to the centre have not received any psychiatric treatment in the past and are experiencing emotional distress associated with social and relationship problems rather than specific psychiatric disorders. The help offered emphasizes family therapy and counselling within an informal non-medical setting.

The Battersea Action and Counseling Centre was established in a deprived inner-city area. Its original objective was to tackle '. . . psychological or interpersonal relationship difficulties whilst at the same time helping the individual to affect his social or envronmental problems' (Holland, 1979, p. 95). Like the other mental health initiatives described here, clients can refer themselves to the entre for help with interpersonal or material problems. The main techniques used are psychotherapy and counseling, but the centre also attempts to respond to the expressed needs of the local population – for example, by setting up a toddler day-care unit to alleviate some of the pressures on mothers in the area. Holland argues that, in some respects, the project has failed to meet its initial objectives. She highlights a number of specific problems including starting, training, funding and the use of volunteers. Two important points – both of which are pursued in the next chapter – are raised; the first relates to the part that a community can bringing about change in their social environment. She argues: 'Good neighbourliness should not be an excuse for the underprivileged to look after themselves on the cheap' (p. 106).

The second point she makes underlines the need to develop mental health services which genuinely involve local people so that they, rather than those who are culturally privileged, predominate.

A rather different project perhaps best represents the way in which initiatives can perform a public health function in more than one area of concern. Although the South Manchester Family Worker Scheme (Spencer, 1987) was established in order to reduce rates of low birth weight in the area, the reduction of psychosocial stress and depression was also considered to be of equal importance.

The project is loosely based on schemes in France which offer women help in the home during pregnancy and after the birth of their baby. The emphasis of the Manchester scheme is the provision of social support, in the form of practical help and advice, to women considered to be at high risk of having a low birth weight baby. Not surprisingly, the factors associated with low birth weight are remarkably similar to those implicated in the development of depression in pregnancy and include lack of emotional support, financial problems, housing problems, and having an unplanned or illegitimate baby (Martin et al., 1982). The Family Workers are selected, not on the basis of formal qualifications, but for their interpersonal skills and own life experiences, The scheme is being conducted as a randomized controlled trial so that it can be properly evaluated. Even though detailed results of the trial are not yet available, early indications are that positive results in both physical and psychological outcomes are being achieved.

The Homemaker Scheme in Glasgow operates on a similar principle to that of the South Manchester project although support is not confined to pregnant women. Families who are having 'problems' are assigned to a worker who will, for example, help around the house, take care of young children, do the shopping or give assistance with benefit claims. The emphasis is on general support with tasks which may be stressful or difficult for the client at that time.

The last example of a community mental health initiative is a Stress Centre which has recently been established in a deprived area of Edinburgh. The idea for the centre came from a group of women who had been meeting regularly in an attempt to reduce and deal with their dependence on tranquillizers (Chapter 8 describes this group in some detail). The Centre is run by the women themselves, there is no appointment system and anyone can drop in at any time for a chat or advice about a problem or difficulties they might be experiencing. It does not have, nor is it run according to, a particular philosophy. It is informal and aims to provide local residents with 'time-out' from their problems as well as practical and emotional support.

The initiatives outlined here have in common the attempt to address mental health problems in the context of the social and material conditions of particular populations. They acknowledge that the antecedents of mental ill health are largely social and that the 'treatments' should therefore incorporate a significant social component – be it in terms of social support, crisis prevention or social change. Mental health initiatives like these, however, cannot hope to effect the major social and environmental hanges which are necessary to reduce mental health inequalities, for example, in relation to the high rates of mental distress and depression among women.

Undoubtedy many womens' lives are especially stressful, the experience of motherhood and childcare bringing particular difficulty and, although the exclusion of many women from the paid workforce after they have children has been identified as one of the main factors related to high rates of depression in this group, it is just one explanation. The sheer number of problems facing some people must surely be a major reason for the observed links between deprivation and depression. Indeed, the fragmentation of disadvantage into its components may actually blur the magnitude of the adversity that many people have to face in their everyday lives and the effect that this has on their psychological well-being. Nevertheless, for those mothers who want it, employment outside the home would not only provide additional income, but would also increase social contacts and eliminate isolation at home. At a time of mass unemployment there are clearly barriers to anyone wishing to gain full-time or part-time employment and it is obviously politically expedient to encourage the view that women should stay at home to care for their children, leaving what jobs there are for the boys. The lack of adequate childcare facilities, however, is an important factor which prevents many women who wish to do so from working outside the home.

Conclusions

The factors associated with poor mental health are – as has already been suggested – not very different from those implicated in physical ill health. As they are largely social rather than individual, many of the solutions must be sought through changes in the social and political environment. Inequalities in resources are going to persist despite political and ideological will on the part of many people. Moreover, even if everyone had good housing, a reasonable income, employment and supportive relationships, pain and distress could not be eliminated and it would be naive to think they could.

Nevertheless, within these realistic constraints there are ways in which inequalities can be redressed and well-being promoted. Provision could be made which would improve the everyday lives of many people.

Public health measures which might promote psychological health are rather different in form, organization and operation from the treatment of mental illness. While the latter is concerned with services for those already suffering from mental ill health, the former are concerned with the prevention and amelioration of the conditions which give rise to disturbance. Psychiatric services are, for the most part, predicated on the assumption that someone only receives treatment once he or she has been defined as a 'case'. Yet, the act of becoming a 'case' through medical and psychiatric referral inevitably distances the individual from the very problems which caused distress in the first place. The way in which mental health services are presently organized and financed largely around hospital and consultant care inhibits the development of community care initiatives which, themselves, could perform important preventive functions.

CHAPTER 8

Promoting Health Through Community Development

Previous chapters have indicated that most physical and mental health problems are more likely to be found in the less affluent members of society and in particular those who live in deprived and disadvantaged areas. These problems are a consequence of fundamental inequalities in the distribution of those resources which can act as buffers against the afflictions of the human condition: good housing, an adequate income, the power, education and money to deal competently with problems, a decent environment at home and work, a life which gives some self-esteem and sense of purpose.

Although personal behaviours such as smoking may be implicated in some diseases and although a poor diet will increase vulnerability to illness, changes in such behaviours are unlikely to occur. This is because the activity itself may be a way of coping with adversity or because of structural barriers to change or, as pointed out in Chapter 5, because the prerequisites for change are not present. Social inequalities in health have so far been resistant to social reforms and changes in health service policy. This chapter outlines one alternative approach to changing the public health and describes an attempt to implement it.

Community Development

According to the *Report of the Royal Commission on the National Health Service* (1979), the first objective of the National Health Service should be to encourage and assist individuals to remain healthy. The now hackneyed phrase, 'the National Sickness Service', is one indication of how far that objective is being fulfilled. Predominantly, activities within the health service focus on acute and chronic hospital cure and care and the assessment of these activities is routinely made by reference to statistics on morbidity and mortality: Thus, it is not surprising that the wider issues of health and illness and their social concomitants remain largely ignored.

As previously indicated, clinical medicine probably plays only a minor role in falling mortality rates and it has been estimated that the medical system affects only about

10% of the usual indices of health and illness (Wildavsky, 1977). It was not these anomalies, however, which led to a change of emphasis in health policy, but rather the escalating costs of health services both in Britain and abroad. As the pattern of diseases changed from one dominated by infectious and communicable conditions to one charac-terized by chronic disorders not amenable to the usual medical armamentarium, the notion of prevention became more important. As indicated in Chapter 1, this was not the preventive emphasis of public health measures, but rather an individualized approach which highlighted the role of personal habits in the aetiology of disease. This position was, of course, influenced by the findings of strong links between smoking and lung cancer. The strength of these findings seems to have also given rise to the notion that other forms of individual behaviour might likewise be of significance, A report from the DHSS (1977b) grounded preventive health action firmly in changes in the attitudes and behaviour of the public and in the encouragement of individual responsibility for health, based upon a regular flow of information and advice from the top down. Health problems were thus seen to inhere in individuals and not in the social structure, in outside agents, or in combinations thereof. This approach was not only naïve but premature in view of the prevailing social, political and economic barriers to the achievement of health by the poorer members of the population. However, it did form part of a movement in health policy which was to press for greater involvement of the general public in health issues.

The Director-General of the World Health Organization in his report to the 28th World Assembly in 1975 recommended a number of principles for successful primary health care, among which were that it should be shaped around the life patterns of the population it was there to serve and should meet the needs of the community. Further, it was recommended not only that primary care should be fully integrated with the activities of other sectors, e.g education, housing and environmental health, but that the local population should be directly involved in the formulation and implementation of health care activities (WHO, 1975). This view was reinforced by the Declaration of Alma-Ata that 'The people have a right and duty to participate individually and collec-tively in the planning and implementation of their health care' (WHO, 1978). Although the idea of public participation in health was hailed as a new strategy it had had its origins much earlier in the community development programmes of the 1960s.

Community development itself has its roots in the colonial programmes of agricul-tural, sanitational and health provision in the Third World, which entailed the organi-ation and support of local people in finding and implementing solutions to the problems they themselves had defined as important. During the 1960s some of the people who had been working in former British colonies, developing skills in community-based work, were returning to the UK and bringing their skills and experience with them. Around the same time UNESCO and other UN agencies were trying to spread ideas and practices relating to the establishment of grassroots projects in Europe. It was hoped to combine the social work techniques used in American poverty programmes with broader developmental work which had had some success in Asia and Africa (Thomas, 1983).

Another important influence, from education, was the work of Paolo Freire. Freire had been directing literacy programmes in Brazil until the military *coup* in 1964 led to his imprisonment and exile to Chile, where he continued to expound his thinking on 'critical consciousness' as a driving force for change, in contrast to attempts to transplant remedies and practices from other cultures. Freire's experiences in South America made him acutely aware of the 'developed' nations cultural invasions of the 'developing' nations. Often there was a conviction about the 'rightness' of the intervention and the benefits it would confer upon the underprivileged. Some parallels with traditional forms of health education will be apparent from the following:

> In cultural invasion the actors draw the thematic content of their action from their own values and ideology; their starting point is their own world, from which they enter the world of those they invade. In cultural synthesis, the actors who come from another world to the world of the people do not do so as invaders. They do not come to teach or to transmit or to give anything, but rather to learn with the people about the people's world. (Freire, 1972, p. 36)

It is this 'learning about the people's world' and the process of 'cultural synthesis' which informs the basic philosophy of community development projects.

It should be noted that increasing divisions in British society between the 'haves' and the 'have-nots' are making the community development approach ever more apposite, with its connotations of validating the experiences and knowledge of another culture.

'The 'discovery' of inner-city deprivation and the fragmentation of communities consequent upon the slum clearances of the 1950s and 1960s began to give rise to serious concern on the part of some government departments and local authorities, although not always from the most altruistic of motives; community development was put forward as one way of tacking the problems of poverty, inequality, sub-standard education and unemployment. In 1969 the Home Office set up twelve Community Development Projects (CDPs) in areas of urban deprivation. It seems likely that at the time the officials concerned with this decision did not fully understand the implications of what they were setting in motion, since community development can he seen as both a philosophy of approach and a programme of action (Du Sautoy, 1966) which incorporates the belief that the ultimate justification for intervention lies not only in the possibility of tangible outcomes, but also in the learning opportunities it provides for the participants, including personal development and the raising of political consciousness.

> Community development is about helping people to reexamine critically the society in which they find themselves, to understand ways in which various political and administrative systems work, to acquire skills in self-organisation and more specific skills that may be relevant to self chosen projects (Baldock, 1974, p. 3).

Longer-term goals are to enhance the interest, competence and participation of marginalized groups in the processes of government. It was predictable that a number of CDPs would develop a radical approach and begin to put forward the view that structural changes in society as a whole were the only real long-term solution for inner-city deprivation. They did this so successfully that government funding was reduced and eventually most of the projects were wound up.

During the 1950s and 1960s a number of trends were operating which produced a new consciousness of health and health issues. The growth of the Women's Movement initiated a challenge to the medical profession and led to a demand for the 'demedicaliz-ation' of women's health and urged women to recover more control over their own bodies. The rapid unionization of health and hospital workers produced new and vocal groupings of people identified with the Health Service, committed to its continuation, but only too conscious of its shortcomings. Community Health Councils were set up in 1974 and began to operate on the principle that improvements in the Health Service could be achieved only through informed dialogue between local communities and those people responsible for planning and policy making. As a consequence some groups who were involved in campaigns to oppose cuts in the health services began to examine more critically the services they were defending and to explore means of improving them.

It was against this background that some of the first neighbourhood health projects employing a community development approach were set up. In 1976, a group called the Foundation for Alternatives, funded six such projects. The Foundation had an advisory committee consisting of assorted academics, general practitioners, health educators and medical consultants and the projects employed community workers whose task it was to explore a community development approach to health education. Some of these projects flourished and others failed, but all of them provided a core of knowledge, information and expertise which provided a basis for future initiatives. At the present time there are about 32 community health projects in England and Wales and 2 in Scotland.

Alongside a growing number of these neighbourhood health projects informal community health initiatives have grown up, such as self-help groups, women's health groups, action campaigns and information and resource centres. The Community Health Information Resource Unit (CHIRU), based in London and funded through DHSS has catalogued thousands of such initiatives all over Britain.

On the whole such activities have taken place outside the National Health Service and in many instances have been a direct result of dissatisfaction with the official response to health needs (Jones, 1983). The scale and diversity of these activities is very great but they share some important characteristics: a collective rather than an individual approach to health; a social rather than a medical model of health and illness; a preventive rather than a curative orientation to health problems. In addition such projects emphasize the participation of the public in health care. When this occurs the focus of attention shifts from agendas of interest to health professionals, such as the cessation of smoking, uptake of screening services, and so on, to a concern with living conditions, inadequate housing, lack of work, feelings of powerlessness and the behaviour of health professionals as the major concerns of lay people at a local level.

Currently most community health projects are funded through charitable trusts, inner city partnership funding or the urban aid programme. Recently, however, Health Authorities and Health Boards have begun to fund small projects, either attaching a community worker to a health centre, group practice or hospital or part-funding interdisciplinary teams of social, health and community workers. The bringing together of these sets of people with their different backgrounds, skills and values has presented the opportunity for breaking down traditional interprofessional barriers, but has also led, inevitably, to conflict. In order to convey the spirit and complexity of community development health projects one such project, located in Scotland, will be described here.

Community Development and Health Promotion in a Deprived Area

In 1984 a pilot project, funded by the Scottish Home and Health Department for 2 years was set up in a deprived housing estate on the periphery of Edinburgh. The objective of the project was to explore ways of involving general practitioners in health promotion in the community and to find means of creating channels whereby people in the community could communicate their health needs and concerns. The experience gained during this pilot phase in creating channels for public participation and in highlighting the problems, dilemmas and strategies for success led to the granting of funding for a further 2 years and the addition of a health visitor and a research worker to the project.

One serious barrier to involving a community in health issues is that, as a rule, community development workers do not have the training or contacts necessary for the inclusion of health issues in their work. Health professionals, conversely, lack the knowledge, training and contacts necessary to the promotion of public participation in health. In particular medical education tends to encourage and reinforce barriers to genuine dialogue between doctors and patients by inculcating the notion of 'expert opinion' in both groups, such that neither places much credence in the validity of the lay perspective. Moreover, the orientation of doctors, health visitors and other health professionals is heavily biased in favour of an individual orientation rather than a community one.

Accordingly it was decided by the management committee during the pilot phase of the project that one way of addressing these problems would be to attach a full-time community worker to a large general practice, in which one of the general practitioners would be funded to work for two sessions a week on the project. In this way it was intended that each would develop an understanding of the other's ideology and practices and that together they would endeavour to involve the local community, other professional groups and local health personnel in a combined attack on local health problems.

Starting off

Prior to tacking the major objectives of the project certain preparatory activities were necessary, for example, becoming aware of and documenting local resources and establishing the organizational base of the project. It was in these early stages that hints of the major problems to come began to be received. The problems encountered were broadly representative of general obstacles to the smooth running of many such projects and will be described later.

Becoming aware of local resources provided by statutory services, voluntary organizations and community-based groups enabled the community worker to draw a basic picture of the different strands of health service and health education provision in the area. This also gave an insight into some of the barriers to genuine interprofessional cooperation, geographical and psychological boundaries, organizational structures and professional values and attitudes. At a practical level it also revealed a wealth of resources which were potentially available to the project; meeting rooms, equipment, funds and possibilities for joint work. In addition, an impression was gained of the social networks that were operating, local boundaries between sub-groups and neighbourhoods, local antagonisms and key people in the community.

Establishing an organizational base was an important task in the initial period. Secretarial help was offered by a community workshop and photocopying facilities by the Social Work department. A small room was provided by a group general practice as an office for the community worker, but there was no telephone or typewriter. As the general practitioners did not wish to give the receptionists any extra work there was no means of relaying messages. Eventually a telephone and an answering machine were installed. In addition, the room provided was located in a 'private' part of the practice to which it was virtually impossible for local residents to gain access. Since, by definition, community development work involves a major commitment to contact and informal interaction with members of the local community, these organizational details were of the utmost importance.

A small survey of residents and local professionals was carried out in order to obtain information about definitions of health, health needs and perceptions of health. In general, professionals tended to define health in broad, abstract terms, such as those adopted by the World Health Organization, incorporating a notion of well-being. Local residents tended to define health in more specific, concrete and personal ways where feelings 'inside' were seen as having paramount importance, closely followed by being happy, feeling energetic and alert. Both groups were asked to define a 'healthy community' and to say what factors affected health. Responses fell into six basic categories:

1 Socioeconomic: an emphasis upon the structure of the local environment, the standard of housing and recreational facilities and services; this category included income level and unemployment.

    'Got to have an adequate income, employment is important'

2 Social cohesiveness: including ideas of neighbourliness and a sense of community spirit.

    'One that talks to each other and listens to what they say.'

3 Personal responsibility: this involved the idea of individuals being less dependent upon services, taking decisions about their own health and being educated to use the services appropriately.

    'A community willing to accept a bit of responsibility.'

4 A medical model: this defined health as freedom from disease.

    'Free of scourges like TB, drug abuse and avoidable disease.'

5 A behavioural focus: here individual behaviour was held responsible for health problems.

    'Smoking and drinking aren't good for your health.'

6 Social support: the divisive or supportive nature of personal relationships

    'Stress in the home affects you.'

This small survey highlighted the different perceptions held about health. There was congruence between people in defining health in practical ways such as being well enough to do the things they wanted to do and in the definition of factors affecting the health of the community, in particular, social and economic factors and the need for social cohesiveness. Health professionals were, however, somewhat more likely to emphasize individual responsibility for personal behaviour as of prime importance in the amelioration of health problems.

Local residents in deprived communities are rarely asked for their opinions or involvement and encouraging active participation is, therefore, a sensitive process, especially when an active dialogue is believed to be more desirable than authoritarian exhortations. One way of initiating this process was to ask local people to help with a survey, to make suggestions about topics that should be covered and to carry out some interviews themselves. In this way the community worker was working alongside local people in beginning to define the health needs of the community. This also helped to raise the interest and awareness of the interviewers in the health issues about which they were gathering information. This, in turn, led to a desire to discuss some issues in greater depth and a women's discussion group was formed around the topics of childbirth and stress. This pattern of involving a small number of individuals in a particular activity and of these people then forming a core which drew in more people through friendships and informal contacts, was one which was successfully repeated throughout the course of the project. As the project gathered momentum further contacts were made and the pressure of work began to build. Since the project had been funded for only 2 years initially, decisions had to be made during the pilot phase about which activities were feasible in the time available. What became increasingly apparent was that members of the community were eager to participate and anxious to find means of addressing their health concerns. The project became more widely known and a variety of individuals approached the community development worker with requests for advice, which indicated the need for a lot of basic information: where to get help for alcohol problems, how to ask for particular childbirth procedures, how to register with a doctor, how to get a health visitor to call, what the action of certain medicines was and what a positive cervical smear meant.

Some people requested help with personal problems for which they had not sought care through the official channels, either because they were frightened or felt alienated or simply because they did not know where to go. Responses to such requests involved providing emotional support, sending out information, helping to write letters to consultants or making suggestions about whom to contact, either a professional or someone else in the community with a similar problem.

It became apparent that for many people contact with health and social services was not a straightforward and satisfactory interaction, but one that left them feeling frustrated, powerless, unskilled, ignorant or unheard. The very act of becoming a patient, a client or a case engendered a sense of passivity and compliance. The social background and training of most doctors creates a significant cultural gap between them and the people they are supposed to serve. In addition, white coats, glass barriers, long corridors and linguistic differences produce an atmosphere which is alienating and intimidating to many of the clientele.

The community worker also made contacts with other workers in the area in order to inform them about the nature of the project and how it might link in to aspects of their own work. Time was taken to visit most of them in person and at least some were interested in the possibility of collaborative work. At intervals, the community worker was invited to speak about the project at team meetings of community education workers, social workers and teachers, as well as, later, health visitors and district nurses. Joint work was undertaken most easily with local community workers perhaps because of the familiarity they had with each other's worlds. Resources from the community education team were made available to fund tutors for sessional work with groups and crèche workers.

Since the project was based in an area where local schools play an active role in community life, teachers, too, were interested in cooperating with the project and help was offered with accommodation, equipment and educational materials, as well as the use of a swimming pool. This led, in the second 2 years of the project, to relocation of the project in a local school, at the invitation of the headmaster.

The local social work team was supportive and one of their workers helped in the early days of establishing a support group for people wishing to reduce their dependency on tranquillizers. The community psychiatrist was interested and gave a number of sessions on mental health to local groups, discussing depression, stress and how to cope.

Contacts were gradually built up with local agencies such as health education, schools and community centres. Links were also made with the Scottish Association for Mental Health, the local Health Council, the Scottish Drugs Forum and the Regional Council's Health Committee. Items in the local newspaper were used to introduce and maintain the focus on the project. A news sheet explaining the project and its purpose, together with the results of the local surveys, was distributed to every household.

Major Activities of the Project

Small groups were formed and met regularly for varying lengths of time, to discuss topics such as women's health, the relationship between health and housing conditions, stress and feeding children a healthy diet. The groups generated alternative means of responding to health needs, e.g. founding a self-help group for people wishing to reduce their dependency on tranquillizers (as already mentioned), forming a compulsive-eating group, the planning of a stress centre, identification of useful information and support for mothers with young children.

Practical activities included the setting up of a pensioners' swimming group and a fruit and vegetable cooperative. Opportunities were created whereby local people and professionals could meet and identify health needs in the community with the aim of encouraging the development of a dialogue between local groups and policymakers at health board level. One example of this was the establishment of an Elderly Forum which is a mix of elderly people and professionals working with the elderly in the area. This forum has made recommendations to the Joint Working Party on the Elderly, set up by the Scottish Office.

Links have begun to develop between all these activities with, for example, a member of the tranquillizers group driving to the market for the fruit and vegetable cooperative, using his own van; and members of the swimming group planning the coming programme of activities and some joining the Elderly Forum. Members of the tranquillizers group are helping to plan the stress centre and two of them are now employed to work there.

Funding was extended for a further 2 years in 1986 and the community worker was joined by the health visitor, whose primary task is to liaise with members of the primary health care team and to engage in group work. A research worker is evaluating the project as a whole. The move to the new site in a primary school enables local people to drop in on a casual basis and provides a meeting point. A part-time administrative assistant who lives locally is also employed.

From the various activities initiated by the project it is possible to give only a few detailed examples, but these should convey the complexity of the various processes such work sets in train.

The women's health discussion group

This group grew out of the interest expressed by two groups of women who were using adjacent buildings – a children's centre and the community centre. The women planned sessions with the community development worker and discussions were held on confidence, stress, the shape we are, sexuality and talking to doctors.

The numbers in the group varied between 8 and 12 each week. A crèche was provided, an essential feature if women with young children are to be able to attend and join in the discussion without interruptions. After the initial programme a core of seven women wished to continue meeting. They focused on damp housing as a topic of concern in relation to health, and over a 12-week period they made a slide-tape presentation entitled Home Sweet Home. The educative component of this enterprise was a prime feature. The women had to organize material, interview people, decide on the questions to ask, prioritize points and assemble a coherent programme on a complex issue. To obtain official information they identified and interviewed professionals such as housing officers, councillors and a general practitioner. They learned about how housing services were organized and who was responsible for the health aspects of housing. This slide-tape presentation was eventually shown at a seminar in Edinburgh University and gave rise to a research study on damp housing and health status. This study established significant relationships between the presence of dampness/mould and emotional problems in adults and a variety of physical symptoms in children (Martin et al. 1987). The findings were used by Edinburgh District Council, Lothian Regional Council and Shelter, amongst others. An important feature of these events is that they illustrate that it is possible for lay people to initiate academic research and to influence research workers to carry out research which is relevant to public need without sacrificing the rigour of scientific method.

Two members of the health group went on to become active in the community. One was a founder member of the tranquillizers group and the other became active in the local tenants group and in a city-wide campaign against damp housing.

Tranquillizers group

The formation and subsequent development of this group provides an example of how people may come together on the basis of a very specific shared need and by meeting that need collectively go on to tackle wider public health issues.

The area of the project is one of high tranquillizer and antidepressant use and the persistent taking of tranquillizers was a major concern of local women. Initially, members needed a lot of support in reducing their intake of drugs and coping with withdrawal symptoms. As their symptoms abated and trust developed, the active role of the community worker changed and group members took on more responsibility for running the group. As each individual gained confidence and began to feel better she or he acted as a role model for the others and for new members. By acquiring skills in relaxation and breathing, building confidence and sharing information about the composition and effects of tranquillizers the group developed both knowledge and self respect. Eventually all the regular attenders were able to relinquish their dependency on drugs. The original members of the group are now in demand to share their expertise with other similar groups; with community organizations, social work students and others. This demand led to acknowledgment by group members that they had important experience and information to share. Accordingly, they applied for funds, adopted a constitution, wrote and published a booklet.

The crucial aspect of the group experience lay in helping people to escape their inner isolation and to move beyond the idea that they had an illness which was their individual problem – a view often exacerbated by medical contact. Despite the growing literature on benzodiazapine withdrawal, many of the group members had been convinced that their withdrawal symptoms were solely a reflection of their emotional problems or personality difficulties and they had no idea that theirs was a common experience. Now, not only has the initial purpose of the group been fulfilled, but the members have become an important community resource for mental health in their own right, developing personal, social and organizational skills in the process. Two of the original members are now employed at a stress centre, set up by local people, to act as a preventive facility.

Food and families group

Mothers in a mother and toddlers group were approached and asked if they would be interested in exploring the idea of food and families over a 5 week period. Between six and eleven women attended these discussions. After an initial period during which they explored the various influences which affect the way children are fed, they decided to make a slide/tape programme which focused on feeding babies and young children. Topics included breast or bottle feeding, help available and introducing solids. The group examined critically the available leaflets and advice received from health visitors and information which did not fit with experience was rejected. By this process the group began to identify specific information they would have liked at particular times in the lives of their children, the type of help they required and ways in which services could be more responsive to their needs. The slide-tape programme entitled Who Knows Best? encapsulates these views in a form which can be used to create and stimulate dialogue between the users and the providers of a service.

Pilton Elderly Forum

The Elderly Forum is an example of the achievement of a longer-term aim of the project – to enhance the participation of marginalized groups in health care planning. After a year's work with elderly people in the area, the establishment of a swimming group and the fruit and vegetable cooperative, a health course and a summer programme of activities, these different strands were pulled together with the help of other community workers and the participants themselves. This culminated in the establishment of the Elderly Forum, which contains a mix of local people and workers. It has been meeting regularly for the past 2 years tackling such issues as the prescribing of generic drugs, chiropody services, labelling of medicines and sheltered housing provision. Many of the issues are difficult to deal with at local level, because they require a shift of policy or attitudes at a higher level. Some necessitate cooperation between professional groups, such as social workers and health service workers – and others necessitate the setting up of a channel of communication so that locally defined needs can be expressed to those engaged in planning health care services.

A Scottish Office circular on Joint Planning led to the setting up of four Joint Working Parties, on mental health, physical disability, mental handicap and the elderly. After the latter had produced its first report it was seeking comment and suggestions. The Elderly Forum was in a strong position to respond to this and 50 pensioners took part in a working day conference, adding their comments and ideas. Recommendations on housing, health services and social work were made, together with practical suggestions for having them implemented at local level.

In this example three elements were in operation which facilitated the participatory process – these were a level of community organization, the joint planning structure and a means of communication between the two. Unfortunately, these elements are not always present coterminously. Community groups often wish to make their views known but cannot penetrate the bureaucratic structure of the health services; progressive ideas initiated at middle or senior management level founder because of an inability to inspire and support workers on the ground. Hunter (1987) has emphasized the need to address and resolve the problems of this nature inherent in Joint Planning, through coordinated action at and between every level of policy-making.

These few examples show the potential that lies within a community development framework. By respecting people's own knowledge and beliefs and using this as a starting-point, some of the problems deprived communities face can become the topic of critical discussion, leading to new and unexpected insights. The discovery of the potential within local residents raises the question of how services can become more responsive to local need and highlights areas where change is needed. It also raises awareness of the health problems that individuals and the community face in everyday life. By providing the opportunity for people to engage in discussion in an informal setting the beginning of a climate is created whereby participation in health care planning could become a reality.

The ultimate aim of the project is that the workers will withdraw and the various activities will be managed and extended by members of the community. To this end an increasing number of local people are being drawn into the project as voluntary or paid workers. The current management committee will gradually be replaced by one formed from local residents.

Evaluation

Since the major initiatives of the 1970s there have been attempts to evaluate community development projects but these have met with little success. This can be explained, in general terms, by the inadequacy of research techniques for evaluating developmental processes. More specifically, where traditional research would rigorously assess how far outcomes match objectives, this is clearly not applicable to community development where the objectives and priorities are continually changing. The application of such strict methodology would distort the very essence of the work. In addition, it must be admitted that some community workers are ideologically opposed to objective evaluative techniques, believing that the work is self-evidently of value. Pampling (1985) has argued that descriptive, analytical accounts are more relevant to projects such as the one described here. Certainly, it is the case that outcomes are often impossible to pinpoint, since most effects have the form of a continuing process. Thus 'snapshot' evaluations can give a misleading impression.

Community health projects of the 1970s relied upon 'critical appraisals' and produced some useful case studies (NCVO, 1979). However, there has been an increasing demand for more rigorous evaluation of projects, not only from funding bodies, but from community workers themselves (LCHR, 1986). As pointed out by Martin (1984) a propos community mental health projects:

> We can say of all these projects that they have admirable intentions and show interesting lines of development, but we are in no position to say unequivocally that they are successful. Success must be judged in terms of beneficial changes achieved in the lives of patients or clients and those around them, and cannot be inferred from statements of aims or even from the use of particular methods, unless the general effectiveness of those methods has been satisfactorily demonstrated. (p. 167)

A paper given by Sommerville (1984) has outlined some of the specific problems of using traditional scientific methods for this type of work, including the difficulty of obtaining control groups, the inability to specify relevant population variables and the fact that measurable health outcomes, such as changes in mortality and morbidity figures may take many years to show up.

The addition of a research worker to the project reported here was intended as a means of tacking some of these issues as well as allowing the presentation of a formal assessment of the worth of the project, together with the identification of those factors which facilitate success or predict failure and under which particular circumstances. The evaluative techniques eventually adopted were chosen in order to test the feasibility of a variety of methods. This is regarded as a first step in identifying valid and reliable indicators of the performance of community development projects in health.

Methods being used include the following:

1 Action research which documents the number and the development of groups, the number of participants in each group, attrition and the reasons for it. Accounts are solicited from members of the groups about their reasons for joining, their experiences in the group and the effects it has on them. Causes of satisfaction and dissatisfaction are documented. Individuals who drop out of groups are interviewed. The information obtained is fed back to the groups themselves and to the workers on the project and the process continues.

2 A survey, carried out by local people, who have been trained in interviewing techniques, gathered base-line data about health status in the community, awareness of health issues, knowledge of local facilities, utilization of primary and preventive services, knowledge of and involvement in the project activities, demographic details and social and environmental problems. This survey will be repeated at intervals throughout the project. Using local people to conduct interviews also has the virtue of putting money into local pockets, raising the awareness of the interviewers about

their own neighbourhood and, incidentally, eliciting highly reliable information since the interviewees find it easier to talk naturally to people with whom they can identify.

3 Routine hospital statistics, use of accident and emergency services and psychiatric admissions are being monitored, as well as health visitor data such as uptake of immunisation.

4 For one week out of every month each of the three project workers keeps a daily diary of activities and comments which is discussed at a regular monthly meeting. The diaries are used to obtain a description of the flow of events, to pinpoint problems, to identify facilitating circumstances or barriers to action and to provide a commentary on the project.

5 A list of people who contact the project is kept, together with reasons for the contact. In this way the widening of the circle of professionals and lay people in touch with the project can be described, together with perceptions of its activities and influence.

6 A quasi-controlled study of parent education is being carried out. This consists of offering all mothers with children under 2 years old one of several parent education experiences, including small group work. As far as possible, those who accept will be randomized to the different strategies and the outcomes compared in terms of increased knowledge and uptake of and demand for services. Mothers who do not accept the invitation will also be included in the study and compared with those who do.

Conflicts and Contradictions

Not all the attempts to establish activities in the community have been successful. Some failed through lack of support, inability to find appropriate facilities, e.g. a room to meet in, or time constraints. The community worker was severely overtaxed for the first 2 years, until she was joined by the health visitor and research worker. It should also be remembered that people who live in a stressful environment can find it difficult to attend regular meetings; crises occur, babysitters cannot be found, illness is a common occurrence. Such factors impose barriers to a commitment to attend meetings on a regular basis.

Experience of the project so far has raised many important issues. Obviously, there was both a need and a desire in the community for participation and a 'voice'. However, structural constraints constituted unexpected obstacles to participation and the project would have benefited from more workers earlier in its development, more facilities and a more accessible base. Its current housing in a primary school has proved to be much more acceptable and local people are able to drop in as and when they wish. In general, however, local people have posed few barriers to the philosophy or strategy of the project. Conversely, the vast majority of problems have arisen from professional attitudes and behaviour and the bureaucratic structures of officialdom. Conflicts and confusions have arisen which are largely a consequence of introducing a community development approach into an area where professional roles and rules are already well established.

Official support from the medical profession and from health boards for community development strategies in health promotion seemed to have grown from a tacit admission that health services were failing to make an impact on the considerable volume of poor health in deprived communities. Health education, too, seemed to have little effect in these areas. Since health services are dominated by a medical model which focuses on individuals as the objects of treatment, the solution to major health problems has been seen to lie in getting members of the public to change their behaviour; to stop smoking, to take up preventive services such as screening, to change their diet and so on. Chapter 5 has suggested that this expectation is quite naïve from a theoretical perspective and Chapter 6 has indicated that the role of individual behaviour in aetiology may be less significant than factors which create a general susceptibility to illness. When health problems are seen to inhere in individuals, rather than being endemic to social structure and circumstances, attention is directed towards short-term solutions only and the conditions which are largely responsible for the problems remain constant.

Thus, the initial and, in some cases, continuing expectations of medical and health personnel with respect to the project were that it would focus upon concerns of interest to them. This is, of course, quite inimical to the principles of community development, which is non-directive and wholly concerned with the perceived needs of the local population. The topics raised by local residents tend to be those which relate to the social and emotional distress in the area. The conflict to which this gives rise can be illustrated by reference to two specific issues.

First damp housing and its effect upon health was an issue about which concern was expressed many times early in the project. It was felt to affect the physical and mental health of both adults and children. Mothers had drawn attention to the recurrent chest and upper respiratory infections which prevented babies and toddlers from completing immunization. The mental stress caused by living in a damp and, often, mouldy house, which defies efforts to maintain a clean place to live, is exacerbated by overcrowding consequent upon having rooms which are uninhabitable. Financial hardships, are compounded because of the need to spend more on heating and damaged furniture. In general, tenants felt themselves to be unsupported by health professionals in this matter.

Most health visitors were sympathetic to tenants' views and confirmed the problems with immunization, but when the women who had made the slide-tape presentation about their housing conditions showed it and asked for their support, it was apparent that the health visitors felt unable to deal with the matter in any way other than as an individual health problem. The general practitioner initiated a discussion with representatives from the local health board, about the system of medical 'lines' for rehousing and it became clear that officers of the board took no account of mental stress when recommending rehousing, since emotional problems were not considered to be a health problem. This is in spite of the fact that two-thirds of letters from general practitioners are concerned with effects on mental health of inadequate housing conditions. There is, thus, a profound difference of opinion not only as to whether housing is a health problem but if it is, whose is the responsibility. There are professional and administrative reasons for health professionals to regard poor housing as somebody else's business, most obviously the local authority's. However in terms of health, housing officials refer to medical professionals to assess its impact. Responsibility for these public health issues, once under the aegis of a Medical Officer of Health has become fragmented since the reorganization of health and social services in 1974. It is ironic that only after the tenants had persuaded some professional research workers to investigate the issue, with the result that the tenants' complaints were vindicated, that housing and health officials began to take notice. Doctors tend to regard housing issues as 'too political' and at a meeting organized by the Regional Council to set up a forum of professionals and local people to tackle the housing and health issue, only one general practitioner out of the eighteen who were invited actually turned up.

The second issue is the local concern with tranquillizer use. Once participants had learned about side-effects, they felt that they had been seriously misled by their doctors and became very critical, both of their General Practitioners and of the psychiatric services they had experienced.

There tends to be an assumption that health promotion requires changes in the behaviour solely of members of the public; however, it is clear that the community development approach also requires fundamental changes in the behaviour of the professional groups who serve the community, such as doctors, social workers and health visitors. Without their support the active participation of the public in decision-making for health care becomes a practical impossibility. Whereas health professionals tend to see their role in health promotion as encouraging a reduction in smoking or adopting preventive measures such as hypertension screening programmes, local people may feel that there are more pressing issues which are affecting their health.

Attempts which have been made to bring public and professionals together on a basis of mutual and equal respect have so far been largely unsuccessful. For example, two general practitioners expressed interest in the tranquillizers group and said they would like to attend a meeting. The community development worker felt it necessary to consult the group before this was agreed to. Some members of the group were patients of the general practitioners concerned, others had expressed resentment against their own doctors and, most importantly, the group belonged to the members and was a place for them to share experiences which were confidential.

The general practitioners, however, were unused to asking patients about their own acceptability and expressed some resentment that they needed the permission of the group before they would be allowed to attend. Few doctors are used to soliciting the approval of their patients. In the event, only one of the doctors met the group and the occasion was not a success. Perhaps because this group was seen as intruding into the area of clinical judgement, it was viewed with suspicion initially, and some GPs indicated that they felt tranquillizer use was not a particular problem, that the group should not cast doubt on their clinical judgement or prescribing habits and that patients should tackle the problem with their doctors rather than their peers. A leaflet was produced in the hope that GPs would refer some patients to the group whom they felt might benefit from the social support to be obtained there. However, the leaflets were rarely used and referrals came from only one woman doctor.

Some of the foregoing problems stem from lack of familiarity with the precepts of community development, from feelings of having professional territory invaded and from anxieties about loss of power, particularly when some of that power is being claimed by the very people over whom it was formerly exercised. Some difficulties can be ascribed to pre-existing internecine rivalries, well known but rarely openly acknowledged, which exist within and between workers in the health and social services. Thus it is necessary to spend a great deal of time educating and motivating professional groups. It is certainly not the norm for doctors and others to relate easily to autonomous groups of lay people.

Other obstacles to cooperation are related to organizational constraints. Community workers are used to dropping in casually to project offices, community flats and community centres, where people work informally and with few hierarchies of rank and power. Entering health centres, group practices, hospitals or health service buildings which are designed to separate the staff from the public by means of appointment systems, glass barriers and uniforms can be daunting and frustrating, not to mention alienating for the clientele.

If support is lacking through ignorance or misunderstanding about community development, those who are involved in the planning and delivery of health services, from medical treatment to health education may find it equally as difficult to give whole-hearted support once they *do* understand the principles upon which it is based. Since the prime objective is to raise critical awareness in members of the public, one inevitable result is a demystification of professional authority and language. Once people have developed awareness of what is affecting their health and the shortcomings of the official services, the 'informed choices' they make may not be the ones preferred by the 'experts'. This represents a significant challenge to the power and expertise of the latter. If intersectoral and interprofessional cooperation are to be achieved, and they are vital to the elimination of deprivation, some fundamental changes are needed in professional beliefs, pride and behaviour. Such changes will include a greater willingness to admit openly the limitations of a narrow focus on individualized treatment; an enhanced appreciation of the advantages of alternative approaches; a desire to cooperate with other groups including members of the public on equal terms; and the development of respect for the knowledge, skills and potential to be found in any community.

An understanding of the reasons behind much of the conflict between doctors, community workers and other health professionals is essential if cooperation is to be maximized. Part of the explanation would seem to lie in the very different socialization experiences of the people involved and part in the clash of 'social realities' which they inhabit.

Mizrahi and Abramson (1985) have analysed some differences between physicians and social workers which are pertinent here, although it should be borne in mind that social workers as a whole have greater cohesion and more structure as a profession than do community workers. In addition, the former work more in a hierarchical and group context. Differences of sex, status, social class and income are also important. Many doctors, either by virtue of training, or by preference, develop an aloof demeanour vis-a-vis patients, possibly because of problems in dealing with the emotions raised by constant confrontations with disease, death and distress (Stein, 1985).

Community workers, on the other hand, tend to place a high value on the expression of feelings and give maximum importance to the establishment of warm and open relationships with local people. Whereas doctors tend to adopt an individual orientation, community workers are alert to the complexity of social circumstances in which people live and tend to see the medical model as trivializing and reductionist.

A busy general practitioner faced with a full surgery tends, perforce, to focus on some available practical intervention, processing patients with little time to discuss or delve far beneath the surface, even when aware of and sympathetic to the wider context of the patient's life. The relationship with the patient, unless he or she is of similar status, will tend to be authoritarian and one-sided. The community worker operating at local level and more constantly in contact with the daily social problems of the people can gain access to complaints about doctors and the health services. Indeed, part of the work will involve documentation of ways in which primary health care services do not meet the needs of the community. This activity is obviously not one to enhance the popularity of community workers with medical personnel.

Letourmy (1986), albeit in the French context, poses the question of why doctors, entrenched in a type of activity which is expected of them, highly valued in society and useful, should take any interest in social inequalities and the social concomitants and causes of ill health; an arena for which they are ill equipped by background, training and, possibly, inclination. Unless a meaningful and convincing answer to this question can be found, there may be little point in berating doctors for actions which are perfectly reasonable from their professional perspective. It may be necessary for community workers to adapt to this situation and by demonstrating the worth of their work hope to convince by example. Douglas (1970) has pointed out that things remain the same in societies because any society tends to support the preferred values it contains. Hierarchical systems such as the medical profession must control information and access and persuade those at the bottom and their clientele to share their values. According to Douglas's analysis the most important rules and values reflect weaknesses in the system. Thus, for the medical profession, with its restricted ability to prevent disease, limited capacity to deal in any meaningful way with many of the problems presented to it and knowing that the majority of patients are either not in need of medical care *per se* or have self-limiting conditions, the need to preserve the notion of having special knowledge and 'magic bullets' is very important. Naturally there are many individual doctors who are sympathetic to the aims of community development, but the fact that community development health projects exist is in itself a challenge to the dominance of the medical profession as a whole.

The recent publication of the *Cumberledge Report* (DHSS, 1986) has led to discussion of ways in which some of these problems of intersectoral cooperation might be addressed. Cumberledge proposed that neighbourhoods of between 10,000 and 25,000 people should establish a nursing service, managed by a nurse and coordinated by health visitors, district nurses, school nurses and, eventually, nurses attached to general practices. In this way some of the professional rivalries and organizational tangles might be sorted out if, as was intended, such a service could provide a basis for more effective cooperation between all health workers in the community with an emphasis on developing services founded in local needs with maximum lay involvement. As such it could be part of a radical public health movement. However, this document is still under consideration and it remains to be seen if its recommendations will ever be implemented.

Claiming ownership of areas of multiple deprivation has become a way for local authorities to attract money, often without any clear idea of how the funds can be used to maximum effect. Twenty years of urban programmes have seen millions of pounds poured into areas, only for most of it to vanish into the bank accounts of developers and others outside the community. In that time the deprivation and despair have only got worse. Sometimes the solution has been seen in terms of sending in yet more 'experts', increasing the number of professionals working in the area. However, sending more professionals into communities already overburdened with the weight of outsiders who come and go without any discernible long-term changes being achieved can scarcely be the answer. Community development principles require that skills and resources are potentiated within the community itself, implying that any available funds should be used to encourage and stimulate local involvement. A major stumbling block has been the tendency of professional workers to take over once significant needs have been identified. One solution to this is for professionals to share their skills and knowledge with local people and for the skills and knowledge of local people to be given credence. The strategy of the project described in this chapter has been to involve local people at all levels beyond that of simply 'articulating needs', e.g. training people to design questionnaires, carry out interviews, code and analyze data; employing only local people to work on project activities; ensuring that local input reaches official channels and, ultimately, handing over the project to the community (if, indeed, the community wants it!).

Further frustrations can arise from the fact that health projects such as the one described here are expected to prove themselves in a very short period of time in ways which are acceptable to the agency funding the project. The expectation that a maximum impact can be achieved with a minimum of investment is unrealistic. Multiple deprivation is the product of decades, sometimes generations, of neglect and exploitation. It is unlikely to be successfully ameliorated in the 2 or 3 years for which most such projects receive support. In addition, the demand that 'desirable' outcomes be demonstrated represents an anomaly in that the public are expected to define their own needs and objectives, but outcomes may be required to reflect official and professional concerns. The strategy of evaluation in the project reported here has been to utilize a variety of the methods as described previously. In this way it is hoped to gather data of interest to professional bodies and also of more direct relevance to the aims and expectations of the community development approach.

Another concern of projects such as this one must be that a focus on health as a major problem in areas of multiple deprivation may lead to fragmentation of the total issue, which is one of poverty and powerlessness. By slanting problems towards individuals and not the social structure in which they live, the amelioration of deprivation is undermined. It should not be forgotten that while individuals come and go from deprived areas, the underlying social conditions which are largely responsible for their excessive amount of ill health remain the same. Before people can be expected to take responsibility for their own health they need to gain some self-esteem, to feel proud of being who they are, to gain control over their lives and to have a decent environment in which to live.

Finally it is important to be aware of the danger of yet another supposedly 'radical' movement being co-opted into the service of the power structure. 'Community' solutions find favour with both major political parties, for, of course, quite different reasons. Encouraging communities to solve their own problems can mean big savings of public money and therefore has a strong appeal to the right side of the political spectrum, as long, presumably, as those solutions are not too disruptive of the status quo. On the left, community participation is hailed as bringing power to the people. The same kind of phenomenon occurs in relation to health promotion as is pointed out in the next chapter.

Bryson and Mowbray (1981), in the Australian context, have called community participation the 'spray-on solution' and everyone is in favour of such democratic initiatives. However, they do imply that the community is willing and able to take on the mammoth task of sorting out problems which are a consequence of mismanagement, carelessness, thoughtlessness or callousness on the part of governments, local authorities and/or big business. There has been vociferous objection, especially in relation to community care, to using members of the community (usually women) as unpaid workers in an 'invisible welfare state' (Waerness, 1978).

It, has been known for over 2000 years that the poor get sick more and in that time, relatively speaking, very little has altered. Community development projects have great potential for bringing about change and there is reason to believe that support for practice can be found in a theory such as that described in Chapter 5. It will, however, take many years before the results can be expected to manifest themselves in ways amenable to traditional forms of measurement or in easily observable ways. Many people are enthusiastic about such projects at the local level. What appears to be needed now is more understanding, cooperation and support from professional and official bodies and some fundamental changes in health and social policy so that community development projects can be accommodated within general strategies for health promotion, without becoming adulterated by institutionalization.

CHAPTER 9

Health Policy and
Health Promotion

Previous chapters have drawn attention to the persistence of social inequalities in health; the minimal impact of traditional medical practice on health status; and the need for fundamental changes in practice and policy. In the last three decades medicine has tended to consolidate its dependency on clinical and high-technology practices. This trend has posed problems to health policy-both in terms of the desirability of such an approach in dealing with the prevailing burden of ill health and in terms of cost feasibility.

In the 1970s the impact of medicine, and of health policy in general, on people's health status and the reasons for a reduced emphasis on caring and prevention, as compared to curing, came under scrutiny. Since that time the literature on these themes has grown and is supported by recent initiatives from the World Health Organization which advocates the need for a 'new' public health strategy with a focus on health promotion.

This chapter will first analyze emerging concepts in health policy. These concepts stem from cost-containment pressures, but also from the changing patterns of disease and from an increased scepticism about the role of medical services in the promotion of the public health. Secondly, it will point out differences between traditional health education and health promotion initiatives. Finally, it will explore some of the major uncertainties in the use of intersectoral decison making as a key requirement for the development of health promotion policy. Chapter 8 focused on the community-based implementation of health promoting measures; the present chapter will therefore concentrate mainly on the macro aspects of policy-making.

New Concepts in Thinking about Health Policy

Analysts of emerging trends and concepts in any public policy tend to refer to existing policy statements, plans and other official documents. These types of data are an incomplete guide to the actual intentions and hidden motives of policy-makers. Original intentions can soon be forgotten or subtly altered over time. Although the term 'policy' implies a purposive course of action, all too often purposes are defined (or rationalized) retrospectively. In this way, they may imply a greater strategic justification than one might infer from analyzing earlier stages of the policy-making process (Hogwood and Gunn, 1984). Furthermore, as Heclo (1972) points out, a policy can consist of 'what is not being done.' Thus, the question of why there is no policy, or why one particular policy measure is implemented rather than another, may be more revealing than any analysis of official records can convey.

It is with this orientation on official policy statements that the present section explores the emergence of 'new' concepts in health policy documents released by governments in the last decade.

In the 1970s, governmental reports in countries such as Canada (Lalonde, 1974) Great Britain (DHSS, 1976; SHHD, 1977) and the USA (US DHEW, 1979) acknowledged the limitations of conceiving health policy as the mere provision of hospital and medical services. These documents reflected a scepticism that provision of such services alone could further improve the health status of the population. The fact that health policy had become increasingly dependent on high-technology medicine and on expensive hospital-based techniques and facilities was considered undesirable on many grounds. The most obvious was its continually increasing cost.

It was not by chance that the pressure for cost-containment became particularly relevant with the lower growth performance of most Western economies of the early 1970s resulting in what is commonly labelled the 'fiscal crisis' of the welfare states (OECD, 1981). Western governments have been much quicker in setting up cost-containment strategies than, for example, dealing with the problem of social inequalities in health or with health-damaging situations such as unemployment and poverty. Thus, for many countries the response consisted merely of cut-backs in health expenditure (Abel-Smith, 1985). A few countries attempted the more challenging task of documenting the nature and magnitude of the limited role of health policy and medicine in the promotion of public health and proposing a different policy orientation.

In April 1974, the Canadian Ministry of National Health and Welfare released a working document entitled *A New Perspective on the Health of Canadians*; often referred to as the Lalonde Report, after Marc Lalonde who was the Minister of Health and Welfare at that time. It was the first government document, in the Western world, to acknowledge that the current emphasis upon a biomedical health care system is not entirely desirable for the enhancement of health, nor particularly relevant to prevention.

The report pointed out that the increasingly high costs of the Canadian health sector were a consequence of the traditional view of approaching health policy, where 'most direct expenditures on health are physician-centred, including medical care, hospital care, laboratory tests and prescription of drugs' (Lalonde, 1974, pp. 11–12).

Attention was drawn to the fact that this expenditure goes almost entirely on treating illnesses which are already manifest. The claim was made that one way of improving the overall health of Canadians would be to give priority to interventions that are not included in the traditional territory of health care: 'there is little doubt that future improvements in the level of health of Canadians lie mainly in improving the environment, moderating self-imposed risks and adding to our knowledge of human biology' (Lalonde, 1974, p. 18).

The Lalonde Report threw light on the debate concerning which elements of health policy were likely to be most effective for the future; as can be deduced from what has already been said, the debate centred on the relative value of curative and caring interventions to improve the health of citizens who were ill, as opposed to the modification of public and personal measures that affect the individual's environment and life style and may prevent the development of ill health. In order to clarify this debate the report outlined a conceptual framework for re-orienting health policy: the 'health field concept' This concept emphasized the importance of four broad elements as important in health. These were: (a) human biology, the genetic inheritance of the individual, the process of ageing and the many complex internal systems in the body; (b) environment, defined as the influences on health which are external to the human body and over which the individual has little or no control; (c) life style, defined as all the individual's decisions which affect his or her health and over which the individual more or less does have control; (d) and health care organization, which consists of the quality, quantity, arrangements, nature and relationships of people and resources in the provision of health care. The Lalonde Report claimed that the bulk of health expenditures has focused on the element of health care organization, yet the major potential for prevention and health promotion is rooted in the other three elements of the health field concept

The individualistic assumptions about health-related behaviour and the very nature of the concept 'lifestyle' embodied in the Lalonde Report have been criticized by many writers (Labonte and Penfold, 1981; Ziglio, 1983). The definition of lifestyle was vague and ambiguous. The influences of socioeconomic factors and their complex interactions on individual behaviours were neglected. Furthermore, the report did not raise the question as to why 'unhealthy lifestyles' have become so widespread within the population.

The report has been widely acclaimed internationally as a turning point in thinking about health policy and a landmark in the emergence of a 'new' public health movement. What is all too often overlooked, however, is that the Lalonde Report was released at a time when there was a 'cost-crisis' debate in Canada, involving both the federal and provincial governments and their fiscal contribution to health care (Ziglio, 1987a). Such a debate concluded in 1977 in a 'block funding' formula: the Established Fiscal Arrangements Act, which tied federal financial commitments to the growth of the Gross National Product (Weller and Manga, 1983; Van Loon, 1980). The emphasis on 'healthy' individual lifestyle, on individual responsibility for health, and on the assumption that individual behaviour can – if backed up by educational measures – resist the powerful social forces acting upon it, can be seen as an attempt to legitimize cost-containment arrangements and, thus, divert attention from social reforms.

A number of papers have pointed out that after the publication of the report, Canadian public policy, in fact, did very little to control environmental risks – including unemployment and poverty (Miller and Edwards, 1982; Buck, 1985). The 'healthy life styles' proposed by the Lalonde Report were, however, backed by governmental financial support for numerous campaigns to modify individual behaviour. However, as Tsalikis (1980; 1984) argued, the Canadian government, both federally and provincially, particularly supported efforts to change habits which conventional morality perceived as faults in the individual such as drinking, smoking and drug addiction. He added that

> while unchecked economic growth is increasingly producing health risks, government and voluntary campaigns concentrate on teaching individuals how to protect themselves against these risks. Moreover, producers and professionals have moved with

full exploitative force to promote all sorts of commodities and services for anyone in pursuit of a new lifestyle from special jogging outfits to behaviour modification programmes for new ways of living. (Tsalikis, 1980, p. 99)

The individualism of modern health problems is reflected in other governmental reports and policy initiatives in western nations. There is no doubt that the Lalonde Report inspired similar policy documents in Britain (DHSS, 1976) and in the USA (US DHEW, 1979). In outlining the British scene, Robertson (1985) pointed out that Scottish and English official documents on preventive strategies were mainly based on attempts to change individual behaviour through health education, support for vaccination programmes, environmental services, and statements on the need for better coordination between health and social work services. However, if one searches for clear policy statements and financial commitment in official documents such as Prevention and Health: Everybody's Business (DHSS, 1976), Priorities in the Health Services: The Way Forward (DHSS, 1977a), or The Health Service in Scotland: The Way Ahead (SHHD, 1977) the picture becomes vague. Policy objectives remain broadly stated in terms of the encouragement of preventive measures and the development of responsible attitudes to health on the part of the individual and the community (Robertson, 1985; Yarrow, 1986).

Although with some differences, Scandinavian health policy documents released in the 1980s also focused on the recommended shift in health priorities and resource allocation supposedly required to deal effectively with the major health problems of the next decade (Grund, 1982; National Board of Health and Welfare, 1985). Swedish documents in particular represented an interesting attempt to bring together perspectives encompassing both health hazards, which result from macro socio-economic factors, and the micro aspects of individual behaviour. Unfortunately, there was no formulation concerning how the two perspectives might relate to each other. These documents also indicated that the 'new' responsibility for health policy was to initiate coordinated action with other policy sectors based on the identification, monitoring and wide reporting of the health impact of public policy and individual behaviour.

Two Broad Scenarios in the Future Orientation of Health Policy

Beneath the rhetorical commitments to the improvement of health often lie ambiguities as to what actually constitutes a policy for the promotion of health. Thus, it is almost impossible not to find governmental documents paying lip service to public health. Policy statements emphasizing prevention and health promotion can have a breadth of appeal: 'to the left it is part of the progress towards a better society where the social ills of capitalism will be diminished, to the right prevention holds out the hope of reduced government intervention' (Allsop, 1984, p. 173). This surface appeal conceals the very real difficulties and uncertainties surrounding policies for health promotion. For example, the prescription of more intersectoral coordination in the name of health is rarely accompanied by clarification on the ways in which intersectoral cooperation can be facilitated. Moreover, the kind of policy-making processes and conflict resolution mechanisms by means of which changes in health-related policies will be brought about are not addressed. In fact, most policies that affect health are not regarded as 'health policy' and fall outside existing health policy-making processes. Current practice at local, regional and national level very often encourages competition and territoriality, sometimes even hidden hostility. Thus, organizational arrangements, such as intersectoral coordination, should also incorporate practical incentives, and perhaps even tactical concessions, to stimulate involvement by various public policy sectors.

Interference with the decision-making processes of large organizations, for instance business corporations, is usually considered undesirable on 'economic grounds', despite the fact that their operations have a direct impact on physical and social environments. It is not surprising, therefore, that Canadian, British and American health policy documents do not envisage the need to control economic development and its impact on physical and work environments, income and price patterns, as key measures in the promotion of health. Indeed, these documents are still very much conceived within health policy dealing primarily with the provision of personal health services. Concern and commitment to public health has changed direction too many times in history and should teach us to have some scepticism when interpreting shifts in policy orientation.

The 1970s and 1980s have already witnessed the delineation of two main viewpoints in the debate on future developments in health policy. Although some overlap exists, since the two sides are not mutually exclusive, the first orientation aims to introduce cost-containment arrangements which are sometimes an attempt to improve the efficiency/effectiveness of existing health services through better management. The second view advocates the introduction of policies and programmes which would make people less dependent on health services, and consists of prevention, self-help and health promotion. In recent years an emerging emphasis on health promotion, although broadly defined, has increasingly been proposed as a new vision for health policy.

In the coming decades, changes in health policy are likely to be dictated either by a defensive response to cost-containment (where the main policy objective is 'savings', though more appealingly rephrased as 'efficiency'), or by a deliberate effort to identify a new health policy orientation which will be more effective in promoting health. The latter scenario implies a need for a shift in health priorities and resource allocation not just confined to the health sector: a task far from being a straightforward one in most Western developed countries. Within the health sector it implies the pursuit of an appropriate mixture of curing, caring, prevention and health promotion which has to come to terms with the internal and external conflicts that any reallocation of resources generates for professional power and organizational control.

A Move Towards Health Promotion: A Departure from Health Education?

Most countries have health education programmes which aim to change attitudes and individual behaviour through the provision of information. Generally speaking, the rationale of health education programmes is to inform people about diseases and their prevention; to motivate people to change their health-damaging behaviour through persuasion; and to help individuals to gain the skills necessary to minimize health risks. Many health education programmes and campaigns in the areas of smoking, drinking, nutrition, the wearing of seat-belts, drug abuse and sexually-transmitted diseases are conceived within this rationale. Chapter 5 has described some of the limitations of such campaigns and their inadequate theoretical and empirical basis.

The World Health Organization (WHO, 1984) defines health promotion as 'the process of enabling people to increase control over, and to improve, their health.' Thus, although health education is an integral part of health promotion, the latter cannot be conceived narrowly within a disease prevention model.

There is little doubt that despite the often rhetorical acknowledgement of the socio-environmental contribution to ill-health, the main thrust of health promotion in practice has been individualistic and confined to health education. The presence of mainly individualistic approaches to health promotion in Western developed countries is not surprising. According to Draper (1986), it has suited the interests of most stakeholders in the health field. It accommodates the medical model of health and disease prevention that has been predominant for decades and allows governments to commit themselves to the health promotion idea without confronting the complex political questions that a more structural approach would imply. On one hand, it is common to find govern-mental reports and policy statements acknowledging poverty, unemployment and other forms of social deprivation and social inequalities as detrimental to health. On the other hand, practice, or even the existence, of non-fragmented policies addressing such problems, is rare. This is not to say that governments do not have poverty relief programmes, welfare benefits for the unemployed or other underprivileged groups, but, as a large literature on social policy confirms, such initiatives usually have a mitigating rather than a preventive function (Townsend, 1979; Blaxter, 1983; Illsley and Mullen, 1985).

The assumption that individual behaviour is the major factor in the contemporary pattern of ill health is increasingly being criticized, as in Chapter 6, for its middle-class bias and victim-blaming tendencies; its adoption as a way of justifying cut-backs in expenditure on health care (Tsalikis, 1980, 1984; Navarro, 1984); its tendency to deflect attention away from socio-environmental causes of disease and illness (Labonte and Penfold, 1981); and, not least, its empirical base.

In analysing the Lalonde Report, Ziglio (1987a) pointed out that the emphasis on 'soft' persuasion-oriented approaches to life style change presents a relatively easy option for government action. It can be argued that to attempt to change individual behaviour through persuasion alone is to take a naïve atomistic view of the position of the individual in society (Robertson, 1985). Individual life style changes are unlikely to occur, at more than a minimum level, without the economic and structural support which is necessary as a foundation for such changes.

A second perspective is, however, gaining influence in academic circles as well as among health workers, policy-makers and communities. This perspective, broadly referred to as 'structuralist', has a societal and environmental orientation. Policies conceived within this perspective may range from attempts to address health-related issues such as social deprivation and disadvantage, to attempts to bring more health considerations into policy areas such as housing, transport, energy and agriculture, in order to make social and economic development more in tune with the promotion of health. In relation to policy-making strategies this perspective includes health advocacy initiatives which would attempt to influence political and legislative reforms; community development actions to promote social change; and intersectoral decision-making in the formulation of public policy. A variety of supportive measures can be used by structuralist-inspired health promotion policies which aim to bring about structural change through social reforms (Ringen, 1979). These measures can include, for example, legislation and fiscal control.

Structural Reforms and Health Promotion

Social and economic structural reforms are necessary to change the environment which negatively impinges on the public health. At the macro level Norway, in the mid-1970s, offered an example of innovation in the formulation of a national nutrition and food policy inspired by a structuralist perspective (Royal Norwegian Ministry of Agriculture, 1975–6). This policy received considerable attention abroad through the analyses of Blythe (1978), Cohen (1980), Milio (1981) and Ziglio (1985; 1986). The major goals of the policy, which was formally presented by the government to the Storting (National Assembly) in 1975 and approved in 1976, can be categorized as follows:

—global goals: to formulate a nutrition and food policy in accordance with the recommendations of the 1974 World Food Conference held in Rome;
—health goals: to encourage healthy dietary habits;
—food production goals: to increase production and consumption of food produced domestically and increase self-sufficiency in food supply; and
—regional development goals: to utilize food production resources fully, especially in the economically weaker areas.

Although there have been serious difficulties in translating the structuralist-oriented formulation of the policy into practice (Helsing, 1986; Ziglio, 1986). the intention to allow diet and health considerations to influence the production, supply and pricing of food is novel and remains unique in Western developed countries. The fact that the formulation of the Norwegian nutrition and food policy considers the global food situation and the links between nutrition and food, health, agriculture policy and socio-economic development is undoubtedly an innovative feature in public policy-making.

In the 1980s the structuralist perspective was reinforced by a major thrust at the European Office of the World Health Organization. Various WHO documents emphasized the necessity of moving beyond the health care system in promoting people's health and reducing health inequalities (WHO, 1984, 1986a). The WHO strategy of *Health for All* attempted, among other things, to force countries to face to what extent they might search for imaginative new strategies in improving health through an emphasis on health promotion and disease prevention (WHO, 1985). The document *Targets for Health for All* for example invites member states to ensure that legislative, administrative, environmental and economic mechanisms provide support and resources for the promotion of healthy life styles and effective participation of the people at all levels of policy-making (WHO, 1985, Target 13). The specific forms that 'healthy lifestyles' and 'effective participation' may take are, however, very thorny issues and, not surprisingly, are left to the interpretation of the member states.

The concept of health promotion has been further refined in the Ottawa Charter for Health Promotion (WHO, 1986a) The charter advocates the building of a health promotion policy which goes beyond health care:

Health promotion policy combines diverse but complementary approaches including legislation, fiscal measures, taxation and organizational change. It is coordinated action that leads to health, income and social policy that foster greater equity. Joint action contributes to ensuring safer and healthier goods and services, healthier public services, and cleaner, more enjoyable environments.

A move towards health promotion, therefore, represents much more than health education and would constitute a radical departure from traditional thinking on health policy.

It would be an oversimplification of reality to conceptualize measures for health promotion only as products of governmental decision-making (WHO, 1987). It is too narrow and often counterproductive to see health promotion policy solely in terms of governmental policies. The circumstances and environments within which people live are the result of governmental action as well as social relations and processes involving a broad range of institutions, groups and individuals. Governments are more likely to act in those situations where political pressures are generated from organized groups lobbying for reforms. Clearly, as described in Chapter 8, this has implications for the role of community participation in health-promoting policies.

Health promotion may be the greatest opportunity open to public health in the years to come; it may also pose the toughest challenges conceptually, politically and programmatically (Tilson, 1984). To avoid rhetorical statements and naïve approaches to health promotion, an awareness of the major difficulties and uncertainties in policy formulation and implementation is essential.

Health Promotion Policy: Challenges and Opportunities

Although the term health promotion is becoming fashionable it increasingly runs the risk of being charged with so many meanings that it could become meaningless (Tannahill, 1985). Health promotion is usually portrayed as being broader in scope than health education and as having more far-reaching goals than traditional health policy. Unfortunately, it is not easy to have clear-cut definitions of what the concept includes and what it excludes. Health promotion as a general 'vision' of a desirable future may be both seductive in the promise it appears to hold and frustrating in the evasiveness of the answers and practical recommendations which it provides.

Although there is consensus on the conceptualization of an 'image', or 'vision', as a driving force for thinking constructively about the future (Polak, 1961; Masini, 1982), very little is known about the dynamics of image formation, shaping and transmission. Amara (1981) notes that:

> We do not know exactly how images affect individual and social behaviour. We do not know why they sometimes lead cultural development and sometimes lag behind it. We do not even know how amenable they may be to study and analysis. Yet images of the future are so central to the progress of society that an understanding of the dynamics of their formation and renewal is essential. (p. 1)

In health promotion where 'egalitarian', 'ecologist', 'environmentalist and 'self-help' images have dominant roles it would be indispensable to learn how to coalesce private and group visions of the futures so that they could become guidelines for collective action. Health promotion policy-making would require, then, the capability to cope with a rich variety of images without the accompanying divisiveness that makes consensus elusive. At the same time there is the need to learn how to link constructively knowledge, image-forming and political action.

In the attempt to propose a conceptual framework for health promotion, the World Health Organization (WHO, 1984) identified five areas for policy action. The first involved a reorientation of health services and changes in public and corporate policies to pursue 'access to health' and reduce health inequalities. The second area was related to changes in the environment, especially at work and at home. The third concerned the stengthening of social networks and social support, and, the fourth, involved action for the promotion of positive health behaviour and appropriate coping behaviour. Finally, information and education to provide the informed base for making health-promoting choices were regarded as essential.

This categorization has the advantage of being general enough to be relevant to the whole span of member states, and yet the limitation of not being specific enough to convey clear messages for action which can be implemented. Indeed, given these five areas, an unlimited list of issues for health promotion can be generated. As an attempt to provide a conceptual framework for health promotion the 1984 WHO document on the *Concepts and Principles* could have been braver. There is, for example, no specific mention of the need to reorientate the nature of market-based economic developments with their dependency on continuous growth and their often health damaging impact on physical and social environments. General appeals to ecology' and 'quality of life' are of little policy relevance if they are not accompanied by specific analysis on, and policy alternatives to, the present nature of the economic categories of production, consumption and distribution as they influence public health.

The political issues involved in promoting health cannot be ignored if credibility is to be enhanced and victim-blaming approaches rejected. The need for health promotion to be credible, globally conceived and specific enough to be acted upon, does not imply that all the questions surrounding its policy development are already answered. An explicit or implicit health promotion policy is the result of human collective action and is bound, therefore, to be imperfect and generate conflicts and contradictions. It is not in the interest of public health to overlook or disregard such uncertainties. An awareness of them is indispensable to the avoidance of health promotion becoming a sort of religion or dogma. For example, although there is a reasonable degree of consensus about how planning and policy-making have tended to evolve in practice, there is no agreement about how these activities ought to be conducted in the pursuit of change and innovation. The two main approaches to public sector policy-making commonly referred to as 'rational-deductive' and 'incremental' – do not satisfactorily lead up to the planning of change and innovation (Wiseman, 1979; Ziglio, 1987c).

Incrementalism, which implies decision-making by 'muddling through', could not bring about change other than of a marginal nature (Dror, 1964). It would then be unlikely that the structural changes required in promoting people's health could be accommodated within this approach. The rational-deductive approach, which rests on a positivistic-inspired analysis of the problem, where a policy tends to be viewed as an essentially static product, would be maladaptive to the spirit of health promotion. This is because of its lack of consideration of political variables, its use of reductionist methods of problem analysis and its tendency to rely heavily on top-down decision-making. Theoretically speaking, a 'mixed-scanning' approach (Etzioni, 1967; Wiseman, 1978) would stand a better chance of success in planning for change and innovation.

This approach incorporates both rationalistic and incrementalist principles. Policy-making is not seen simply as a rigid goal-oriented process, as in the rationalistic approach. Political considerations and different interest groups are included in mixed-scanning decision-making but, in contrast to incrementalism, it affords wide scope for fundamental decisions and change. Unfortunately, no such approach is as yet well established in the area of health promotion.

An effective move towards health promotion necessitates fundamental changes in traditional ways of considering public policy and its impact on people's health. There is a vast literature on the fact that many policy sectors overlook the health impact of their decisions and, even when an acknowledgement of this exists, health is not necessarily the prime concern in policy formulation. Examples are policies related to farming, energy, transport, economic development and defence.

Lack of knowledge of the health hazards caused by policy decisions in these areas can hardly be considered as an explanation of this state of affairs. In the UK, for example, the work of Draper and his colleagues provided a classification of diseases, accidents and health risks based on the economic categories of production, consumption and distribution (Draper et al, 1977). In the USA the seminal work of Milio (1976; 1977; 1983) analyzed the effect on health of various public sectors, and more recently (Milio, 1983) concentrated on alternative policy decisions which could improve the health promotion potential of public policy over the current situation. Intersectoral planning was seen as essential for developing new and more effective policies with an ecological slant in order to address both macro-economic and public health issues. In Canada the work of Hancock (1980; 1982) provided a new vision for health policy and further evidence for the view that many contemporary illnesses and deaths are rooted in the nature of our energy-intensive and competitive society. Also in Canada, Valaskakis and his colleagues (1981) focused on possible scenarios for economic development and analyzed the environmental impact of a chosen development path. They provided a conceptual framework, based on the notion of a 'conserver society', for changing the current decison criteria regulating economic policy.

In the pursuit of health promotion objectives some mechanisms for intersectoral decision-making are commonly advocated to be desirable both nationally and locally as one of the prerequisites for policy-making (WHO, 1985; 1986a; 1986b). What is not always clear is the magnitude and nature of the obstacles to the adoption of health criteria in public policy decision-making within an intersectoral framework. For example, there is very little critical awareness in the literature advocating intersectoral decision-making of its inbuilt tendency to reach compromise and accommodate diverging interests. This tendency can often be beneficial as it avoids presentation of issues in a 'black and white' manner, allowing policy-makers more scope for manoeuvre. On the other hand, the nature of the compromise can sometimes diminish the credibility of the policy measures adopted which cannot be 'neutral', e.g. the use of educational measures only.

To set up intersectoral committees, or other organizational devices, is not enough. It is necessary to distinguish between the formal aspect of intersectoral decision-making, which can be very impressive on paper, and what actually happens in practice. Intersectoral cooperation can result in yet another routinized bureaucratic device without efficacy and application. Political and bureaucratic boundaries may severely restrict intersectoral decision-making. Political and bureaucratic decision-making is more often motivated by competition for establishing control over decisions, than by a power-sharing attitude which would be desirable in an intersectoral approach.

In Western developed nations, doubts arise as to the political feasibility of the intersectoral approach, and this is particularly true when too much emphasis is put on the role of market forces as the unique mechanism in shaping policy processes and outcomes. There is ample evidence that the assumptions upon which the free market ideology operates e.g. the assumption that the individual exerts a 'free' choice in the market and that his choice is an objective indicator of personal preference and, on a larger scale, of collective inclination – are a distortion of reality (Robbins, 1978).

A closely related issue is the ethical acceptability of local or national interventions, educational, legal and fiscal, aimed at changing individual behaviour, whether by persuasion or coercion. All government decisions and legislation are related to an implicit ethic. The general ethical problem associated with the role of governments relates to how far governmental interventions should attempt to affect the life style of individuals. In pluralistic societies the fear is that certain policies or governmental interventions might erode an individual's freedom to choose (Johnson, 1976).

The distinction between, 'positive freedom' (or 'freedom for') and 'negative freedom' (or 'freedom from') made by Berlin (1975) helps to illuminate the issue. In the area of health promotion one should be sceptical about adopting doctrines based on the concept of negative freedom (i.e. freedom from governmental intervention). Such residualist doctrines are normally justified through the famous claim made by Mills (1909):

> In all the more advanced communities the great majority of things are worse done by the intervention of government, than the individual most interested in the matter would do them, or cause them to be done; if left to themselves people understand their own business and their own interests better, and care for them more, than the government does. (p. 947)

The above statement can be criticized because it implies the 'freedom' to make decisions in isolation from the social and economic conditions in which people live, and ignores the fact that the power to exercise such freedom is constrained by access to economic and other resources which are distributed unequally within society (McCloskey, 1965; George and Wilding, 1976). Nevertheless, in recent years, residualist approaches to social policy have been resurrected in several Western countries – the UK and USA, in particular. On the one hand, residualist approaches to individual and social welfare imply a reduced role for state intervention, a reliance on market forces and an emphasis on the privatization of services. On the other hand, health promotion objectives would largely require a substantial state involvement, legislatively, financially and in the provision of welfare services. This contradiction lacks full acknowledgement.

In developing health promotion policy, governments and other institutions have a fundamental responsibility for the creation of a supportive environment within which individuals can make more easily choices for the maintenance and improvement of their health if they wish to do so. Thus, the concept of 'positive freedom' would better fit a conceptualization of health promotion not limited to an emphasis on mere individual responsibility for health. The problem, however, is to strike a balance between public and individual responsibility and action for health. Thus, in using educational, regulatory or fiscal policy measures, awareness of the dilemma for individual liberty must be recognized, in order to avoid moving into an ideology which rigidly prescribes what individuals should do, how they should behave and in which environment they should live.

Intersectoral Decision-Making and Professional and Organizational Behaviour

The rationale for the decision-making behaviour and attitudes of policy-makers which influence the context within which people's lives are set has very rarely been studied. For example, much of the behavioural emphasis in health promotion focuses on the ways in which the lay public can change (or not change) their attitudes, skills and behaviour. Organizational, professional and policy-makers' attitudes, knowledge and behaviours are usually overlooked – although they may have greater impact in deter-mining the range of choice for individual decision-making and lifestyle.

Organizational and professional behaviours can act as counterforces to intersectoral action at least on three grounds. First, decision-makers and professionals working in government departments, and other governmental or non-governmental agencies, generally tend to squeeze out the maximum short-term gains in each position they hold as they move through organizations (Amara, 1977). In so doing they frequently sacrifice important long-term goals which are fundamental in health promotion. It has been pointed out that many ministries and senior officers like a 'strong department', confusing size and formal power with effectiveness (USHP, 1978). Very often, government depart-ments fight for power rather than for a cooperative solution to complex problems which come within their jurisdiction.

Secondly in intersectoral decision-making, organizational and professional behaviour would imply that a non-hierarchical and participative planning process be one of mutual learning (Trist, 1979; Emery, 1977; Friedmann, 1976). The roles of organizational and professional behaviour in learning processes deserve attention and perhaps also some scepticism. The behaviour of decision-makers working in different organizations should be scrutinized from at least two angles: professional knowledge and expertise; and risk-taking attitudes and behaviours.

As far as the use of professional knowledge and expertise is concerned, this may allow experts and policy-makers to exercise a certain degree of control over some of the factors influencing the promotion of health. Bearing in mind the uncertainty present in this area, e.g. the unpredictability of the impact of the policy measures to be adopted, there must be an awareness of what planners and policy-makers do not know. Ideally, in mutual learning processes such an open confrontation of uncertainty should make it possible to keep the issue of what still remains to be investigated on the agenda. This could indeed lead to new discoveries and innovative actions. However, open confrontation of uncertainty can be used by some departments, or vested interest groups, in lobbying activities based upon what is not yet known, with the intention of stopping proposed health-promotion measures (Ziglio, 1987c). A typical example is the difficulty associated with adopting a price policy – for instance, by means of food subsidies and VAT compensation – aiming at reducing certain nutritionally undesirable consumption patterns and increasing desirable ones. Interest groups such as some sectors of the food industry usually lobby their case on the ground that insufficient knowledge is available to justify policy action.

Risk-taking is another important characterisitic of organizational and professional behaviour. In any policy area, there is no a priori guarantee that the approach chosen will not be disrupted by conflicts in values and solutions held by planners, policy-makers and the public. The saying that 'success has many a father; failure is an orphan' may indeed be applied to most policy decisions. It has been noted (Eaton, 1980) that politicians like to be seen to plan carefully, but they also wish to be protected from blame when a plan fails to meet with public approval. It may happen that, in this latter case, the policy-maker claims to have simply been misled by planners or professional experts. Thus, it seems that advocating intersectoral action and mutual learning must go hand in hand with major changes in policy-making processes and in the willingness to take and share risks and contend with the consequences. This is a very radical departure from the prevailing practice in organizational behaviour and public policy-making in general.

Finally, the pursuit of change and innovation in political processes is, very often, handicapped by a well-documented inability on the part of institutions to promote change or to adapt effectively to it (Crozier, 1969; Amara, 1977). New organizations are often created without dismantling old ones, often resulting in an overlap of functions and a blurring of jurisdictions. Moreover, the structure of many organizations often conflicts with their stated aims and functions. Eide (1981) has argued, for instance, that professions in the social sector (including health) have been fairly satisfied with the limited scope of their policy instruments, as long as their professional dominance within their own sector is respected. Professionalization and institution-building have thus tended to become policy objectives in themselves, usually reducing the beneficial effects of social policies for the ultimate clients. Hence, if the control of institutions has become vested in people who have achieved positions of power, resistance to change may increase proportionately. Our understanding of innovative ways of structuring organizations, so as best to fulfil their goals, is still rather primitive in the public sector (Friedmann, 1976). The tendency towards centralization and pyramidal structures with a vertical chain of command is typical of public bureaucracies. These organizational structures are not necessarily the most effective for coping with innovation (Robertson, 1983). In addition few adequate measures of social accountability exist for judging, and influencing, organizational and professional performances.

In the development of policies for the promotion of health the problems explored in the last sections have to be recognized and addressed at both the formulation and implementation stages. As far as organizational and professional behaviours are concerned, the reliance on managerial change and organizational reforms does not automatically modify possible counterforces to innovation, as the impact of the various managerial and organizational reforms of the British National Health Service have demonstrated (Draper and Smart, 1976; Hunter, 1980). Furthermore, the features of organizational behaviour outlined above do not necessarily apply only to large bureauc-racies such as the National Health Service; community development projects might also develop some of the same resistance to change.

Conclusion

Other chapters in the book have given close attention to the context of people's lives, the role of social structure in inequalities in health, and the influence of the media in imposing particular views of reality. As far as the objective of promoting health is concerned, social and economic factors- normally considered to be beyond the purview of traditional health policy- have a direct impact both on people's health and on the conditions within which individual and collective action takes place.

Policies for the promotion of health need to integrate the issue of health into a wider social, economic and political context. This complexity cannot be handled within the narrow framework which characterizes most of current public policy-making. More imaginative and constructive policy-making needs to be employed nationally and locally. In this respect, the role of health policy which has been traditionally confined to a rather narrow set of mainly reactive measures, often trying to repair the consequences of other policy sectors, has to be changed both conceptually and organizationally. Such a change has to be accompanied by a challenge to the conventional premises of economic development thinking. Thus, a consideration of both short – and long-term impacts on health and well-being has to be increasingly incorporated in the shaping of social and economic policies.

CHAPTER 10

Health, Behaviour and Policy: Towards a Healthy Public

In this final chapter some of the themes which have emerged in the course of writing this book are brought together and some suggestions made for changes in the areas of research and policy in public health. Four issues will be addressed: critical aspects of a focus on lay behaviour; the creation and 'ownership' of social and health problems; research agenda and the way forward to a changing public health.

The Focus on Lay Behaviour

It would be absurd to argue that the habits and activities of individuals have no effect on their tendency to develop diseases. What is problematic is the delineation of the precise role played by behaviour in aetiology, since a theoretical basis from which to test hypotheses is wholly lacking. As previous chapters have suggested, a disease-specific risk factor model has only modest predictive value and then only under highly circumscribed conditions. Conversely a non-specific model which proposes that agents such as bacteria, viruses and carcinogenic substances give rise to disease only once people have become susceptible, *can* account for the fact that similar social variables are constantly associated with many different disorders. Increasing vulnerability due to biological factors, such as ageing, also fits this model, as does the evidence for death and disability following fundamental upsets such as the death of a loved one (Parkes, 1969) or relocation of the elderly (Lieberman, 1961; Aldrich and Mendkoff, 1963). It is also clear that the same agent, e.g. smoking may be implicated in a variety of disease processes and that the same disease, say lung cancer, can be the outcome of a variety of antecedent pathways. In fact, very little is known about the precise role of so-called 'unhealthy' behaviours in the complex series of processes which culminate in diagnosed disease.

In addition to the theoretical, there are a number of practical and ethical difficulties associated with elevating individual behaviour to prime place in the aetiology of disease. Even if some behaviour were of critical importance and even if the majority of people in a given population could be persuaded to change their habits, the impact on morbidity and mortality rates would probably be quite small as not all the people who change their behaviour would have been 'at risk' in the first place. For example, it could be argued that the majority of people who make dietary changes in the direction of lowering their intake of animal fats belong to groups who are the least likely to need to do so. Moreover, new people take on behaviours as fast as other people give them up. A further distinction can be made, in terms of both efficacy and ethics, between influencing individuals who are *known* to be at risk, such as a very heavy drinker who might usefully change or modify his intake of alcohol, and persuading whole groups of people to change in the hope of preventing disease in a few individuals. Finally, the focus on individual behaviour diverts attention from what may be more appropriate and efficacious targets, such as bad housing and hazardous working conditions, poverty and poor education. By transferring the responsibility for health problems to individual members of the public, other crucial factors remain largely unexamined.

Professional and political behaviour, for example, in its impact upon the health status of communities, regions and the population as a whole, is largely neglected. Political decisions, however, directly and indirectly influence the context of human lives, the amount of strain which is imposed upon adaptive capacities and the opportunities for well-being. Low social class, deprivation, disadvantage are merely proxy terms for the absence of power, prestige, higher education, comfortable work situations, state subsidies in the form of tax relief on mortgage or other loans, decent housing, financial security, easy access to care and so on, all of which are, at some level, related to political behaviour. Professional workers, whether medical, administrative or in social services, may also behave in ways which are detrimental to the health of the public. These take many forms, from refusing to consider damp housing as a risk to health and, therefore, inappropriate as grounds for rehousing, to the overprescription of drugs for the elderly, indifferent or obstructive treatment of claimants for social benefit or a more general concern with professional issues rather than the purpose for which the profession is supposed to exist in the first place.

The decisions made by industrial companies also affect the lives of thousands of people. The economic consequences of a factory closure, the use of poor-quality building materials, the disregard of the already lax regulations governing the discharge of chemicals into the water and the air, the strain associated with low wages and an uncertain future, may all have significant repercussions for the public health. As Navarro (1975) has pointed out vis-à-vis corporate interests, trying to influence individual food consumption irrespective of the ability of individuals to obtain and purchase more nutritious food ignores the tremendous power of corporate manufacturing industries in determining consumption and their role in the stimulation of demand for particular types of products. There have, of course, been some criticisms of manufacturers of food, tobacco and alcohol for their part in creating and maintaining a demand for 'harmful' products and lobbying governments to intervene by making policy decisions which would affect profits (Jacobson, 1981; Navarro, 1975). However, such criticisms also have the drawback that they too tend to legitimate the focus on individual behaviours.

There exists a curious phenomenon: when there is insufficient or equivocal information available concerning the possible contribution of some set of circumstances to health, whether or not this doubt enters the domain of 'public facts' seems to depend upon the advantage of concealment or revelation to vested interests. For example, a recent survey has indicated that almost 90% of people in a Scottish town have made changes in their eating habits which relate to the publicized risk factors for heart disease (Amos et al., 1987). However, the controversy and doubt which attends these so-called risk factors is scarcely known to the general public at all. Conversely, the difficulty of 'proving' a link between radiation leaks from nuclear power stations and cases of leukaemia and cancer has been the object of many public pronouncements and has been used to justify the continuation of current standards and practices. It is a medically-accepted fact that ionizing radiation is oncogenic and it could be argued that the evidence for environmental radiation as a health hazard is probably much greater than the evidence for diet. The power of commercial and governmental interests to control information and determine policy has been described by Urquhart (1987) in relation to the Dounreay Planning Inquiry, a part of whose task was to assess the evidence that the power station was associated with clusters of childhood leukaemia cases in the vicinity. By deploying a disproportionate amount of time and money and adopting an adversarial style, the authorities were able to dismiss significant data without appropriate consideration being given to it. Urquhart concluded that:

> In the absence of a better method of deciding major planning issues, what is required is a means of constraining the worst abuses of the adversarial process. A start could be made by limiting the vast disparity in the resources available to those participating in planning inquiries. What will be more difficult to achieve is an improved method of publicly assessing expert evidence which does 'not leave participants with the impression that outcomes depend . . . on the skills of advocacy. (p. 26)

Official bodies such as the Health Education Council, when it existed, and the various health education departments of Regional Authorities, have paid scant attention to such issues as river and coastal pollution, damp housing or unemployment and yet the public have as much need of information about the health risks of these conditions as they do about excessive smoking and alcohol use. Exercise has received an unwarranted amount of attention for its supposed beneficial effects, whilst car-driving is rarely seen as problematic behaviour although it is a major cause of death and disability in younger age groups and contributes to air pollution, noise levels and energy wastage.

The Creation and Ownership of Social Problems

The ability of powerful groups to influence debates on matters affecting the public health and to direct attention to some issues rather than others can be seen as part of the process of the social construction of 'problems'. The origin of issues regarded as problematic in a society can be traced to the activities of certain groups acting collectively to establish that some set of circumstances constitutes a problem and then initiating attempts to relieve, change or eliminate the said problem. As Kitsuse and Spector (1975) have suggested; 'what is in contention throughout the social problems producing process are the definitions of reality that groups and organizations assert, sponsor, impose, reject or subvert' (p. 593). It has been observed that it is common for those groups who can be said to 'own' a problem, in the sense of having brought it into being, to try and place responsibility upon other groups to acknowledge the problem as belonging to them and to behave accordingly (Gusfield, 1975). One way in which this is done by powerful groups-government departments, large corporations – is through the transmission and control of 'public facts'.

Farrant and Russell (1986) have documented the ways in which scientific evidence can be translated under pressure from vested interests, political, medical and commercial, to purvey a particular message to the public. The public facts concerning the aetiology of disease, for instance, have undergone social processing so that they now convey the impression that individual behaviour is the major *cause* of health problems. This focus is legitimated by the content of the media, it has become part of official doctrine and the activities of official bodies assert and reinforce this version of reality (Blumer, 1971).

In an analysis of the politics of alcoholism, Weiner (1980) identified the processes by which a problem is (a) animated, by introducing the idea to the public, imparting relevant information and advice; (b) legitimized by official recognition, e.g. in the pronouncements of government ministers and by data-gathering activities; and (c) demonstrated to be a big problem by an escalating number of research reports and papers, the frequency of comment in the media, the setting up of committees and the availability of public money for its investigation. Eventually, a whole array of departments, research establishments, agencies and workers begin to establish territory, claiming parts of the problem as their own and competing for money.

The more the public facts are asserted and reinforced the more apparently obscure and irrelevant opposing evidence begins to seem. Conditions which earlier public health reformers regarded as clearly implicated in disease causation, such as housing and working conditions, have now lost credibility in the eyes of professionals and have been kept on the periphery of the public consciousness. Scientific data are filtered on their way to the public domain and subjected to distortion, selection and suppression in such a way as to make a nonsense of the term 'informed choices'. Abel-Smith (1976) remarked that the main feature of the health market is the consumer's lack of knowledge. This relative ignorance is a feature of the public's dependence upon the gate-keepers in the channels of communication between research workers and the public, whether these gate-keepers be journalists, health educators or government employees. This is also shown in the way in which medicine remains firmly in the public mind as the rightful and principal activity in health care and prevention. Cochrane (1972) wrote of the 'layman's uncritical belief' in the medical profession. Even now, despite the growing popularity of 'ecological' views of health, doubts about medical omnipotence and complaints of insensitivity, few people question the right of doctors to have the dominant voice in matters pertaining to health. Pill and Stott (1982) observed that the medical profession has played a major part in encouraging the belief that it can solve any problem, such that it has itself created a significant barrier to the interest of the public in preventive measures, whether at individual or at population level. The media, too, reinforce this belief with fictional offerings and by over-simplified and adulatory documentaries. In this way public health has come to 'mean' changing individual behaviour. To some extent this processing of information may be regarded as inevitable. The issue thus becomes that of attempting to redress the balance, by tapping into the channels through which information flows into the public domain, by making scientific data more accessible to the public and by ensuring that alternative perspectives are kept alive.

Research Agenda

Current research efforts in health promotion have been criticized throughout this book. Of course, it is far easier to identify the deficiencies of past research efforts than to provide workable alternatives. In this section some aspects of research needs are described.

The bulk of research is largely influenced by two factors: the availability of funding and current thinking on a particular topic. Often these two factors will be related. Because some behaviours are believed to be closely linked to specific health outcomes, research funding has been forthcoming for studies which are specifically focused, e.g. smoking behaviour and cancer, diet and heart disease. Along with smoking and diet, drinking patterns and physical activity patterns are highly researched areas. Most behavioural research currently carried out continues to assess these 'holy four' and accepts the necessity for doing so. Other individual behaviours which take up much time in daily routine, such as driving, shopping, and watching television, are rarely measured or included in studies even though a case could be made that they might have profound effects on the health of people. Thus researchers have emphasized a rather limited selection of possibly relevant behaviours.

With respect to individual behaviours there nevertheless remains a need to understand how these are distributed in the population, how they change over time, what causes them to change and what constitutes evidence that they have changed. A theory which moves away from emphases on individual cognitive processes and introduces a societal, contextual component was presented in Chapter 5. There is, however, clearly a need for competing theories of behavioural change which incorporate both organizational and individual behaviour which can be tested and accepted or rejected. Assessing what has 'caused' or brought about any behavioural change will probably remain illusive until this more basic research is carried out. However, just as it is unlikely that specific diseases can be attributed to only one specific causal factor, so it is unlikely that behaviours and behavioural changes can be pinned down to single triggers. It seems more probable that a variety of antecedent factors will be involved. This so-called problem of 'attribution' has stymied health education research; the issues will not be resolved by short-term research projects, nor by single-discipline researchers, but by long-term, multidisciplinary, multicentre research commitments.

Despite the extraordinary documentation of some health-related behaviours there is relatively little information about how these behaviours relate to one another in populations. This is not simply a measurement problem, but is recognizably promulgated by the manner in which much behavioural research is funded. The wider concept of health, championed by health promotion, that a healthy life style, incorporating numerous health-related behaviours, leads to a *general* outcome of better health appears to have a limited constituency within those agencies and organizations which allocate resources for research.

Throughout this book it has been argued that behaviours, individual, professional and organizational, occur in a context. This may take many forms but is generally conceived of as socioenvironmental. While it seems intuitively obvious that behaviours occur in some setting, e.g. the family, it is remarkable how seldom research on health behaviour probes into this context, although there are, of course, exceptions. With respect to drinking behaviour, there is an extensive literature on where the drinking takes place, with whom and why, as well as broad ethological studies of the cultural context of drinking. But this literature is unusual and most health-related behaviours are usually measured without reference to the context of daily life. Furthermore, many behaviours thought of as being harmful to health may well be indulged in, not through ignorance, but through choice, either in the context of coping with the exigencies of daily life or as part of conscious and pleasurable indulgences. There is a need for more research to cover these positive aspects of 'negative' health behaviours.

Another area which is relatively untapped is the relationship of changes in health-related behaviour to the perceived health status of the individuals concerned. There is some evidence that the cessation of smoking often has no noticeable effects on health and may make some people feel worse (Hunt and MacLeod, 1987). The taking up of regular exercise may also give rise to unpleasant aches and pains. The strain, physical and mental, which may ensue upon behavioural changes may in itself increase general susceptibility to illness or give rise to compensatory behaviours of unknown effect. This also bears investigation.

The preoccupation of most behavioural and social scientists with individual lay behaviours has left a large research vacuum with respect to organizational and professional behaviour. There is, of course, a rich tradition of organizational research, particularly on health care organizations, but this has generally been isolated from behavioural research which has emphasized individual behaviour. The need for dialogue between these two 'levels' of research, the one assessing micro (individual) behaviour, the other macro (organizational) behaviour, needs to be fostered. It is probably clear to many behavioural scientists that the two levels are synergistic, but by what mechanisms is an important area of study. Chapter 8 drew attention to the way in which professional behaviour can facilitate or impede strategies for health promotion and this is a seriously neglected area of research. The term 'health behaviour' should thus be seen to incorporate the behaviour of health professionals, administrators and policy-makers.

Influencing Policy

It cannot be denied that, for the most part, research has had only a limited impact on changing the public health. Why this has been and remains the case represents an important research need in itself. In his extensive review of the literature on the use of research, Karapin (1986) states:

> Social scientists are frustrated that their work is not used as they think it should be, and dismayed that they do not share the social esteem of natural scientists. Sometimes this situation may endanger research funds. With their economics in trouble, nations like the US and Britain have begun to decide that social science is an expendable luxury. As a result the 'under-utilisation' of research has received a surge of new attention, although the field has already had citations increase fifty-fold in the twenty years preceding 1976. (p. 236)

e0 Utilization of research needs critical attention; on that there is wide agreement. Having said that, the relevant literature appears to have several problems. First there is the usual difficulty of definitions and measures of utilization. Secondly a powerful prejudice against 'positivism' characterizes much of the literature although this has, in turn, resulted in efforts to develop an 'action research' paradigm which emphasizes local knowledge in contrast to the application of universal laws in specific cases (Susman and

Evered, 1978). Thirdly, utilization research has often emphasized the empirical, descriptive research over the theoretical (Bulmer, 1982). As Karapin (1986) again reports:

> Research conducted or sponsored by the British government is firmly in this empiricist tradition; descriptive, factual, statistical and not very theoretical (p. 245).

There are a number of other reasons why research may have had such little impact on policy. First, it may be a consequence of the narrow interests of the researchers themselves who perceive their remit to end with the publication of their findings in a 'respectable' journal. Secondly, when researchers do adopt a more aggressive stance, they tend to prefer rhetoric to action and to preach to the already converted. When it comes to a contest between career prospects and a moral stance there is little doubt about the outcome. This is particularly the case in a climate of cutbacks, shrinking prospects and competition for funding. Much important research which links social conditions to ill health is tucked away in scientific journals, the language and location of which limit any impact it might otherwise have. The distribution of significant research findings directly to the people concerned and to sympathetic policy-makers in a language free of jargon and padding would be surely more effective; certainly it could not be less so than at present. It should be borne in mind that the bulk of research into health matters is sponsored directly or indirectly by government bodies, councils, or commercial interests, or initiated at the whim of high-ranking academics.

It is rare indeed for the public to have a say in the content or direction of research studies even though they are the subjects of it and largely pay for it, although there are precedents (Martin et al., 1987). Moreover, much of the reported research has focused on 'linkages' between policy-making and evaluation research. Studies concerned with identifying sources of influences, whether they be organizational governmental, media-based or the public itself, and linking these sources to properly conducted evaluation research are required. Nevertheless, such endeavours are not without their critics (Casanova, 1981; Weiss, et al., 1982). It is not, therefore, necessary to abandon the empiricist, positivistic tradition. Nor is such an approach incompatible with an 'action' orientation. Each should and could inform the other and, in doing so, may have more influence on policy.

Recent developments in health promotion research which have been discussed in earlier chapters have identified the use of research as a central theme in health promotion. Furthermore, this book has emphasized not only the needs for further research but also the great amount of extant research which could or should lead to an improved public health. Thus the challenge is to put this research into a context where it will lead to an improved public health. This implies, as Gustavsen (1986) has termed it, a 'participative dialogue' between researchers and the people to whom it pertains. Beyond that it implies a broader 'dialogue', perhaps a forthright communication between those who sponsor research and those who carry it out. This presumes a spirit of compromise and communication among all parties. How to bring about this communication needs to be given a high priority on the research agenda.

The Way Ahead

The behavioural and social sciences are in a time of transition. The establishment of multidisciplinary research units to conduct research into health, behaviour and change is an example of an organizational response to the research needs. On a larger scale, initiatives such as the WHO Research Action Plan for Europe, and the concerted action research programmes of the Medical and Public Health Research Committee of the Commission of the European Communities, are examples of efforts to respond to the changing public health needs of the industrialized West.

Many would argue that health education has a very limited impact on the public health. Health promotion, to date, has either comprised the strategies and practices of health education under a new name or has consisted of much rhetoric and little action. The adoption of a health promotion policy by a government does not necessarily imply anything about implementation of such policies; nor does it ensure a change in the public health. It may well be that a reliance on the benevolence of governments to create policies which will encourage intersectoral cooperation and put controls on the health-damaging behaviours of industrial organizations, is simply naïve.

What may be more feasible is the setting up of alliances between public and professionals at grassroots level, particularly in deprived communities. Chapter 8 has described some activities along these lines and has shown that such cooperative enterprises can be successful in bringing pressure to bear on policy-makers at local and regional levels. Such an alliance could include lay people, doctors, academics, lawyers, research workers and health professionals. They would act collectively to highlight local problems (which would in all likelihood have relevance for other communities), initiate relevant research where more information was needed, feed that information to local people, official bodies and the press and lobby for action to be taken in a concerted manner. Subsequently, the processes and outcomes related to the action could be evaluated.

Professional groups need to be more vocal in redressing the current imbalance in the health information reaching the public. A letter to the *Guardian* expressing outrage at some state of affairs is likely to be much less effective than a few minutes on local radio, an article in the community newspaper or a personal appearance talking to local people. In addition, health professionals and research workers can help demystify medical practice. They can share skills and funding with deprived communities, e.g. by passing on techniques for the critical analysis of information, research design and data collection and involving local people in surveys and problem definition. There is a need for people who live in disadvantaged areas to see that positive changes can be brought about by individual and collective action in the community and in the workplace. Helping this to occur is just as much a public health activity as is the provision of clean water or encouraging the uptake of preventive services. Experts could thus become resources for the community.

There has been a tendency by most members of the medical profession and by many social scientists working in the health field to eschew 'politics'. However, health and disease *are* political issues, simply because they are profoundly influenced by political decisions and power relationships. Controversial issues too often turn out to be those that threaten vested interests, one of the abilities of which is to define what shall be regarded as controversial.

Virchow (quoted in Rosen, 1979) wrote:

> that very word Public Health shows those who were and still are of the opinion that medicine has nothing to do with politics the magnitude of their error (p. 62).

There can be little doubt that an adequate income, decent housing, a clean environment and a range of coping skills are key elements in the prevention of ill health. However, the view that all these will come to pass if only we strive for even greater economic growth is increasingly seen as a limited perspective. What is needed is a better appreciation of the relationship between policy and health. Health objectives need to be built into all policy decisions as part of a basic needs strategy, so that departments responsible for energy, defence, transport, food and agriculture, and employment would automatically assess the impact of their policies on health. In the last analysis, a generally healthy public requires fundamental changes in political and professional behaviours, change that is much more likely to influence the public health than giving up butter or taking up jogging, but which will require a new commitment to human well-being.

Conclusion

Although we have often taken a critical stance with respect to current public health efforts it is, of course, easier to find the weaknesses of a paradigm than it is to create a new one. Nevertheless, it is through criticisms of contemporary assumptions and traditional models that a synthesis and a move towards more appropriate ideas can be promulgated. There is widespread dissatisfaction with many of the approaches to understanding factors related to health, but at the same time there is a sense of urgency around the development of practical and theoretically sound research strategies for improving the public health. It is clear that many of these strategies must centre on the amelioration of deprivation and disadvantage and the influencing of public policies concerning social and environmental issues. Only when this has been achieved will significant advances have been made towards changing the public health.

References

Abel-Smith, B. (1976). *Value for Money in Health Services*. Heinemann Educational Books, London.

Abel-Smith, B. (1985). Who is the odd man out? The experience of Western Europe in containing the costs of health care, *Milb. Mem. Fd. Quart.*, **63**, 1–17.

Abel-Smith, B., and Titmuss, R. M. (1956), *The Cost of the National Health Service in England and Wales*, Cambridge University Press, Cambridge.

Abrams, D., Elder, J., and PHHP staff (1981). *Pawtucket Heart Health Program: General Theoretical Model*, Pawtucket Heart Health Program Technical Report, Rhode Island.

Achinstein, P. (1968), *Concepts of Science: A Philosophical Analysis*, John Hopkins Press, Baltimore, Md.

Adelstein, A., MacDonald-Davies, I., and Weatherall, J. (1980), *Social and Biological Factors in Infant Mortality 1975–6*, Office of Population and Census Surveys, HMSO, London.

Adler, M. W. (1981). Medicine and the media, *BMJ*, **283**, 1395.

Ajzen, J., and Fishbein, M. (1980). *Understanding Attitudes and Predicting Social Behaviour*, Prentice-Hall Inc., Englewood Cliffs, NJ.

Aldenderfer, M. S., and Blashfield, R. K. (1984). *Cluster Analysis*, Sage, London.

Alderson, M. (1966). Referral to hospital among a representative sample of adults who died, *Proc. Roy. Soc. Med.*, **59**, 719–21.

Aldrich, C. K. and Mendkoff, E. (1963). Relocation of the aged and disabled: a mortality study, *J. Am. Geriat. Soc.*, **11**, 185–94.

Alexander, F. E., O'Brien, F., Hepburn, W., and Miller, M. (1987). The association between mortality rates and socio-economic factors for G. P. practices in Edinburgh: an application of small area statistics; unpublished paper.

Allport, G. (1961). *Pattern and Growth in Personality*, Holt, New York.

Allsop, J. (1984). *Health Policy and the National Health Service*, Longman, London.

Alonzo, A. E. (1979). Everyday illness behaviour: a situational approach to health status deviations. *Soc. Sci. Med.*, **13A**, 397–404.

Alonzo, A. E. (1984) An illness behaviour paradigm: a conceptual exploration of a situational adaptation perspective, *Soc. Sci. Med.*, **19**, 499–517.

Alwain, D. F., and Hauser, R. M. (1975). The decomposition of effects in path analysis, *Am. Soc. Rev.*, **40**, 37–47.

Amara, R, (1977). The future field: functions, forms and critical issues, in *The Study of the Future: An Agenda for Research* (ed. W. I. Boucher), Government Printing Office, Washington DC, 46–62.

Amara, R. (1981). For tomorrow: images, institutions, involvement, *World Fut. Soc.*, November–December, 1–4.

Amos, A. (1984). Women's magazines and smoking, *Hlth Ed. J.*, **43**, 45–50.

Amos, A., Currie, C., Hunt, S. M., and Martin, C. (1987). Health-related behavioural change in relation to age and sex; unpublished paper.

Anderson, R. (1983). How have people changed their health behaviour? *Hlth Ed. J.*, **42**, 82–6.

Anderson, R. (1984). Health promotion: an overview, *Eur., Monog. Hlth Ed. Res.*, **6**, 1–76.

Anderson, R. (1986). Research on health behaviour: an overview; paper presented to World Health Organization Symposium on Health Behaviour: Its Application to Health Promotion,

Pitlochry, to be published in *Behavioural Research in Health Promotion* (provisional title) (eds. R. Anderson, J. K. Davies, I. Kickbush and D. V. McQueen), Oxford University Press, Oxford.

Andrews, G., and Tennant, C. (1978). Being upset and becoming ill: an appraisal of the relation between life events and physical illness, *Med. J. Aust.*, **1**, 324–7.

Aneshensel, C. S., Frerichs, R. R., and Huba, G. J. (1984). Depression and physical illness: multiwave, nonrecursive causal model, *J. Hlth Soc. Behav.*, **25**, 350–71.

Anon. (1980a). An appalling Panorama, *BMJ*, **281**, 1028.

Anon. (1980b). Invincible arrogance – and patients suffer, *BMJ*, **281**, 1509–10.

Antonovsky, A. (1967). Social class, life expectancy and overall mortality, *Milb. Mem. Fd. Quart.*, **45**, 31–8.

Arber, S. (1987). Social class, non-employment and chronic illness; continuing the inequalities in health debate, *BMJ*, **294**, 1069–73.

Asher, H. B. (1976). *Causal Modeling*, Sage, London.

Askham, J. (1975). *Fertility and Deprivation*, Cambridge University Press, London.

Atkinson, J. M. (1971). Societal reaction to suicide; the role of coroners' definitions, in *Images of Deviance* (ed. S. Cohen), Penguin, Harmondsworth, 165–91.

Bach, F. F., Duval, D., Dardenne, M., Salomon, J. C., Tursz, T., and Fournier, C. (1975). The effects of steroids on T cells, *Transpl. Proc.*, **7**, 25–30.

Bachrach, K. M., and Zautra, A. J. (1985). Coping with a community stressor: the threat of a hazardous waste facility, *J. Hlth Soc. Behav.*, **26**, 127–41.

Backett, E. M. (1975). Domestic accidents, World Health Organization Public Health Paper, No. 1, Geneva.

Backett, E. M. (1977). Consumer detriment in health, in *Why the Poor Pay More* (ed. F. Williams), National Consumer Council, London, 93–129.

Backett, K. C. (1987). The achievement of health: the middle classes discuss health in families, Research Unit in Health and Behaviour Change Working Paper No. 13, Edinburgh.

Baird, D. (1974). Epidemiology of low birthweight changes in incidence in Aberdeen 1948–1972, *J. Biosoc. Sci.*, **7**, 77–97.

Baird, D. (1975). The changing pattern of human reproduction in Scotland 1928–1972, *J. Biosoc. Sci.*, **6**, 322–41.

Baldock, P. (1974). *Community Work and Social Work*, Routledge & Kegan Paul, London.

Bandura, A. (1969). *Principles of Behaviour Modification*, Holt, Rinehart & Winston, New York.

Bandura, A. (1979). The self system in reciprocal determinism, *Am. Psychol.*, **79**, 144–58.

Banks, M. H., and Jackson, P. R. (1982). Unemployment and risk of minor psychiatric disorder in young people, *Psychol. Med.*, **12**, 789–98.

Barker, D., and Osmond, C. (1987). Inequalities in health in Britain: specific explanations in three Lancashire towns, *BMJ*, **294**, 749–52.

Bartley, M. (1985). Coronary heart disease and the public health 1850–1983, *Soc. Hlth Ill.*, **7**, 289–313.

Bauley, B. R., Johnson, M. R. D., Bland, J. M., and Murray, M. (1980). Trends in children's smoking, *Comm. Med.*, **2**, 186–9.

Baum, A., Fleming, R., and Reddy, D. M. (1986). Unemployment stress: loss of control, reactance and learned helplessness, *Soc. Sci. Med.*, **5**, 509–16.

Bebbington, P., Hurry, J., Tennant, C., Sturt, E., and Wing, J. K. (1981). Epidemiology of mental disorders in Camberwell, *Psychol. Med.*, **11**, 561–79.

Becker, M. H., Haefner, D. P., Kasl, S. V., Kirscht, J., Maiman, L., and Rosenstock, I. M. (1977). Selected psychological models and correlates of individual health-related behaviours, *Med. Care*, **15**, 27–46.

Belson, W. A. (1986). *Validity in Survey Research: With Special Reference to the Techniques of Intensive Interviewing and Progressive Modification for Testing and Constructing Difficult Measures for Use in Survey Research*, Gower Publishing Aldershot, Hants.

Benfari, R. C., Eaker, E., and Stoll, J. G. (1981). Behavioural interventions and compliance to treatment regimes, *Ann. Rev. Pub. Hlth*, **2**, 431–71.

Berkman, L. F., and Breslow, L. (1983). *Health and Ways of Living: The Alameda County Study*, Oxford University Press, New York.

Berkson, J. (1962). Mortality and marital status, *Am. J. Pub. Hlth*, **52**, 1318–21.

Berlin, I. (1975). Two concepts of liberty, in *Self-determination in Social Work* (ed. F. E. McDermott), Routledge & Kegan Paul, London, 141–53.

Best, G., Dennis, J., and Draper, P. (1977). *Health, the Mass Media and the National Health Service*, Unit for the Study of Health Policy, Guy's Hospital, London.

Birkett, D. P. (1988). Colon Cancer: the emergence of a concept, in *Medical Aspects of Dietary Fibre* (eds. G. A. Spiller and R. M. Kay), Plenum Medical Book Co., New York, 75–81.

Blackburn, H., Luepker, R., Kline, F. C., *et al.* (1984). The Minnesota Health Program: a research and demonstration project in cardiovascular disease prevention, in *Behavioural Health: A Handbook of Health Enhancement and Disease Prevention* (eds. J. D. Matarazzo, S. M. Wiess, J. A. Herd *et al.*), John Wiley & Sons, New York, 1071–104.

Blair, S. N., Collingwood, T. R., Reynolds, R., Smith, M., Hagan, R. D., and Sterling, C. L. (1984). Health promotion for educators: impact on health behaviours, satisfaction and general well-being, *Am. J. Pub. Hlth.*, **74**, 147–9.

Blalock, H. M., Jr (1964). *Causal Inferences in Non-experimental Research*, University of North Carolina Press, Chapel Hill, NC.

Blalock, H. M., Jr (1968). Theory building and causal inferences, in *Methodology in Social Research* (eds. H. M. Blalock and A. B. Blalock), Mcgraw-Hill, New York, 155–98.

Blalock, H. M., Jr (1969). *Theory Construction: From Verbal to Mathematical Formulations*, Prentice-Hall, Englewood Cliffs, NJ.

Blane, D. (1985). An assessment of the Black Report's 'explanations of health inequalities', *Soc. Hlth Illn.* **7**, 423–45.

Blaxter, M. (1981). *The Health of the Children: A Review of Research on the Place of Health in Cycles of Disadvantage*, SSRC/DHSS. Studies in Deprivation and Disadvantage, 3, Heinemann Educational Books, London.

Blaxter, M. (1983). Health services as a defence against the consequences of poverty in industrialised societies, *Soc. Sci. Med.*, **17**, 1139–48.

Blaxter, M., and Paterson, E. (1982). *Mothers and Daughters: A Three Generational Study of Health Attitudes and Behaviour*, Heinemann Educational Books, London.

Bloor, M. (1978). On the routinised nature of work in people-processing agencies: the case of adeno-tonsillectomy assessments in ENT out-patient clinics, in *Relationships between Doctors and Patients* (ed. M. Alan David), Saton House, Farnborough, Hants, 38–52.

Bloor, M. and Horobin, G. (1974). Conflict and conflict resolution in doctor – patient interactions, in *A Sociology of Medical Practice* (eds. C. Cox and A. Mead), Collier Macmillan, London, 271–84.

Blumer, H. (1971). Social problems as collective behaviour, *Soc. Probs*, **18**, 306–17.

Blythe, C. (1978). Norwegian nutrition and food policy, *Food Policy*, **3**, 163–79.

Boddy, F. A. (1983). A report on the work of the unit 1982–3', Social Paediatric and Obstetric Research Unit, University of Glasgow, mimeo.

Bonnano, J. A., and Lies, J. E. (1974). Effects of physical training on coronary risk factors, *Am. J. Cardiol.*, **33**, 760–4.

Borg, G., and Linderholm, H. (1975). Effects of physical conditioning on perceived exertion and working capacity, *Reps. Inst. Appl. Psychol.*, Report No. 63, University of Stockholm.

Boucquet, D., and Curtis, S. (1986). Socio-demographic variation in perceived illness and the use of primary care: the value of community survey data for primary care service planning, *Soc. Sci. Med.*, **23**, 737–44.

Bouras, N., and Brough, D. I. (1982). The development of the Mental Health Advice Centre in Lewisham Health District', *Health Trends*, **14**, 65.

Bourdieu, P. (1984). *Distinction: A Social Critique of the Judgment of Taste*, Routlege & Kegan Paul, London.

Bradburn, N. M., and Sudman, S. (1981). *Improving Interview Method and Questionnaire Design*, Jossey-Bass, London.

Bradley, B. A., and Brooman, P. M. (1980). Panorama's lost transplants', *Lancet*, **2**, 1258–9.

Bradley, J. V. (1968). *Distribution-free Statistical Tests*, Prentice-Hall, Englewood Cliffs, NJ.

Brehm, J. (1966). *A Theory of Psychological Reactance*, Academic Press, New York.

Brennan, M., and Little, V. (1979). Housing and health: recognition of the relationship between housing conditions and population health, *Med. in Soc.*, **15**, 8.

Brennan, M. E., and Lancashire, E. (1978). Association of childhood mortality with housing status and unemployment, *J. Epidem. Comm. Hlth*, **32**, 28–33.

Brodbeck, M. (1959). Models, Meanings and Theories, in *Symposium on Sociological Theory* (ed. L. Gross), Harper and Row, New York, 273–403.

Brotherston, J. (1976). Inequality: is it inevitable? The Galton Lecture 1975, in *Equalities and Inequalities in Health* (eds. C. O. Carter and J. Peel), Proceedings of the 12th Annual Symposium of the Eugenics Society, 1975, Academic Press, London, 73–104.

Brown, G. W. (1974). Meaning, measurement and stress of life events, in *Stressful Life Events: Their Nature and Effects* (eds. B. S. Dohrenwend and B. P. Dohrenwend), John Wiley & Sons, New York, 217–43.

Brown, G. W., and Birley, J. (1968). Crises and life changes and the onset of schizophrenia, *J. Hlth Soc. Behav.*, **9**, 203–14.

Brown, G. W., and Davidson, S. (1978). Social class, psychiatric disorder of mother and accidents to children, *Lancet*, **1**, 378–80.

Brown, G. W., and Harris, T. O. (1978). *Social Origins of Depressions: A Study of Psychiatric Disorder in Women*, Tavistock, London.

Brown, G. W., Nibhrolchain, M., and Harris, T. O. (1975). Social class and psychiatric disturbance among women in an urban population, *Sociology*, **9**, 225–54.

Brown, R. (1965). *Social Psychology*, The Free Press, New York.

Brown, S. (1976). Issues related to developing criteria for the evaluation of risk reduction, *Proceedings of the 12th Meeting of the Society of Prospective Medicine*, Academic Press, New York, 66–70.

Brownell, K. D., Heckerman, C. L., and Westlake, R. S. (1979). The behavioural control of obesity: a descriptive analysis of a large scale programme, *J. Clin. Psychol.*, **35**, 864–9.

Brunner, D., Altman, S., Loebl, K., Schwartz, S., and Levin, S. (1977). Serum cholesterol and triglycerides in patients suffering from ischemic heart disease and in healthy subjects. *Atherosclerosis*, **28**, 197–204.

Bryson, L., and Mowbray, M. (1981). Community: the spray-on solution. *Aust. J. Soc. Issues*, **November**, 255–67.

Buck, C. (1985). Beyond Lalonde – creating health, *Can. J. of Pub. Hlth.*, **76**, (Suppl.), 19–24.

Budd, J., and McCron, R. (1981). Health education and the mass media: past, present and potential, in *Health Education and the Media* (eds. D. S. Leathar, G. B. Hastings, and J. K. Davies), Pergamon, Oxford, 33–43.

Budd, R. W. (1964). Attention score: a device for measuring 'newsplay', *J. Quart.*, **41**, 259–262.

Bull, N. L., and Barber, S. A. (1985). Food habits of 15–25 year olds II: Living accommodation and social class as factors affecting the diet. *Health Visitor*, **58**, 9–11.

Bulmer, M. (1982). *The Uses of Social Research: Social Investigation in Public Policy-making*, Allen and Unwin, Boston and London.

Butler, N. R. and Alberman, E. D. (eds.) (1969). *Perinatal Problems; The Second Report of the 1858 British Perinatal Mortality Survey*, E. & S. Livingstone, Edinburgh.

Byrne, D. S., Harrison, S. P., Keithley, J., and McCarthy, P. (1986). *Housing and Health: The Relationship between Housing Conditions and the Health of Council Tenants*, Gower, Aldershot, Hants.

Callahan, E. (1980). Alternative strategies in the treatment of narcotic addiction: a review, in *The Addictive Behaviour* (ed. W. R. Miller), Pergamon, New York, 217–59.

Calnan, M. (1985). Maintaining health and preventing illness: a comparison of the perceptions of women from different social classes; unpublished paper, Health Services Research Unit, University of Kent.

Calnan, M., and Johnson, B. (1985). Health, health risks and inequalities: an exploratory study of women's perceptions, *Sociol. Hlth Ill.*, **7**, 55–75.

Calnan, M., and Rutter, D. R. (1986). Preventive health practices and their relationship with socio-demographic characteristics, *Hlth Educ. Res.*, **1**, 247–53.

Cameron, D., and Jones, I. G. (1985). An epidemiological and sociological analysis of the use of alcohol, tobacco and other drugs of solace, *Comm. Med.*, **7**, 18–29.

Cannell, C. F., Miller, P. V., and Oksenberg, L. (1981). Research on interviewing techniques in *Sociological Methodology: 1981* (ed. E. Leinhardt), Jossey-Bass, San Francisco, 389–437.

Carpenter, J., Aldrich, C. K., and Bovermand, H. (1968). The effectiveness of patients' interviews: a controlled study of emotional support during pregnancy, *Arch. Gen. Psychiat.*, **19**, 110–12.

Carrington, P., Collings, G. H., Jr, Benson, H., Robinson, H., Wood, L. W., Lehrer, P. M., Woolfolk, R. L., and Cole, J. W. (1980). The use of meditation relaxation techniques for the management of stress in a working population, *J. Occup. Med.*, **22**, 221–31.

Carroll, J. B. (1953). *The Study of Language*, Harvard University Press, Cambridge, Mass.

Carstairs, V. (1981). Multiple deprivation and health state, *Comm. Med.*, **3**, 4–13.

Carter, C. O., and Peel, J. (1976). *Equalities and Inequalities in Health*, Academic Press, London.

Cartwright, A. (1979). *The Dignity of Labour*, Tavistock, London.

Cartwright, A., and Anderson, R. (1981). *General Practice Revisited: A Second Study of Patients and Their Doctors*, Tavistock, London.

Cartwright, A., and O'Brien, M. (1976). Social class variations in the nature of general practitioner consultations, in *Sociology of the National Health Service* (ed. M. Stacey), Monograph No. 22. University of Keele, Staffs, 77–98.

Cartwright, A., and Patterson, P. E. (1966). Distribution of hospital patients by social class, *Hlth Bull.*, **XXIV**, July.

Cartwright, D. (1949). Some principles of mass persuasion, *Hum. Rels.*, **2**, 253–7.

Casanova, P. G., (1981), *The Fallacy of Social Science Research; A Critical Examination and New Qualitative Model*, Pergamon, New York and Oxford.

Cassell, J. (1976). The contribution of the social environment to host resistance, *Am. J. Epidem.*, **104**, 107–23.

Centre for Agricultural Studies (1978). *National Food Policy in the United Kingdom*, University of Reading, Centre for Agricultural Studies.

Champlin, S., and Karoly, P., (1975). Role of contract negotiation in self-management of study time: a preliminary investigation, *Psychol, Rep.*, **37**, 724–6.

Chave, S. P. W. (1984). The origins and development of public health, in *Oxford Textbook of Public Health, Volume I: History, Determinants, Scope, and Strategies* (eds. W. W. Holland *et al.*,), Oxford University Press, Oxford, 3–19.

Ciminero, A. R., and Doleys, D. M. (1976). Childhood enuresis: considerations in assessment, *J. Pediat. Psychol.*, **4**, 17–20.

Cobb, S. (1976). Social support as a moderator of life stress, *Psychosom Med.*, **38**, 300–14.

Cobb, S., and Kasl, S. (1977). *Termination: The Consequences of Job Loss*, US National Institute for Occupational Safety and Health, National Technical Information Service, No. PB282–991.

Cochrane, A. (1972). *Effectiveness and Efficiency*, Nuffield Provincial Hospitals Trust, London.

Cochrane, A., and Moore, F. (1981). Death certification from the epidemiological point of view, *Lancet*, **October**, 742–3.

Cockburn, C. (1977). *The Local State – Management of Cities and People*, Pluto Press, London.

Cockcroft, A. (1982). Post-mortem study of emphysema in coalworkers and non-coalworkers, *Lancet*, **2**, 600–4.

Cohen, C. I., and Cohen, E. J. (1978). Health education: panacea, pernicious or pointless? *New Eng. J. Med.*, **299**, 718–20.

Cohen, M. H. (1980). *Norwegian Nutrition and Food Policy*, Foreign Agricultural Economic Report No. 157, Department of Agriculture, Economic Statistics and Cooperative Science, Washington D.C.

Cohen, R., Appelt, H., Olbrich, R., and Watzel, H. (1979). Alcoholic women: treatment by behaviour-oriented therapy: an eighteen month follow-up study, *Drug Alc. Dep.*, **4**, 489–98.

Cohen, S., and Young, J. (1976). *The Manufacture of News. Social Problems, Deviance and the Mass Media*, Constable, London.

Cole Hamilton, I., and Lang, T. (1986). *Tightening Belts*, London Food Commission, London.

Coleman, J. S. (1964). *Introduction to Mathematical Sociology*. Free Press, Glencoe, New York.

Coleman, J. S. (1968). The mathematical study of change, in *Methodology in Social Research* (eds. H. M. Blalock and A. Blalock), McGraw-Hill, New York, 428–78.

Coleman, J. S. (1973). *The Mathematics of Collective Action*, Aldine, Chicago.

Coleman, J. S. (1981). *Longitudinal Data Analysis*, Basic Books, New York.

Coleman, J. S. (1986). Social theory, social research, and a theory of action, *Am. J. Sociol.*, **91**, 1309–35.

Colley, J. R. T., and Reid, D. (1970). Urban and social class origins of childhood bronchitis in East and West, *BMJ*, **2**, 213–15.

Colley, J. R. T., Douglas, J. W., and Reid, D. (1973). Respiratory disease in young adults: influence of lower respiratory tract illness, social class, air pollution, *BMJ*, **3**, 195–8.

Collins, E., and Klein, R. (1980). Equity and the National Health Service: self-reported morbidity, access and primary care, *BMJ*, **281**, 1111–15.

Comaroff, J. (1978). Medicine and culture: some anthropological perspectives, *Soc. Sci. Med.*, **12B**, 247–54.

Combs, B., and Slovic, P. (1979). Newspaper coverage of causes of death, *J. Quart.*, **56**, 837–43, 849.

Community Projects Foundation (1983). *Community Development and Health Issues: a review of existing theory and practice*. Community Projects Foundation, Edinburgh.

Comstock, G. W., and Hesling, K. J. (1976). Symptoms of depression in two communities. *Psychol. Med.*, **6**, 551–63.

Connell, F. A., Diehr, P., and Hart, L. G. (1987). The use of large data bases in health care studies, in *Annual Review of Public Health* (eds. L. Breslow, J. E. Fielding and L. B. Lave, Annual Reviews Inc., Palo Alto, Calif). **8**, 51–74.

Cook, D., Bartley, M., Cummins, R., and Shaper, A. (1982). Health of unemployed middle-aged men in Great Britain, *Lancet*, 5 June, 1290–4.

Cook, T. D., and Campbell, D. T. (1979). *Quasi-experimentation: Design and Analysis Issues for Field Settings*, Rand McNally, Chicago.

Cook, T. D., and Gruder, C. (1978). Meta-evaluation research; an overview, *Eval. Quart.*, **2**, 5–49.

Cooley, C. (1902). *Social Organisation*, Scribner's, New York.

Cornwell, J. (1984). *Hard Earned Lives: Accounts of Health and Illness from East London*, Tavistock, London.

Costello, C. G. (1982). Social factors associated with depression: a retrospective community study, *Psychol. Med.*, **12**, 329–39.

Court Report (1976), Fit for the future: Report of the Committee on Child Health Services. Comnd. 6684. HMSO, London.

CPE (Community Projects Foundation) (1983). *Community Development and Health Issues: A Review of Existing Theory and Practice*, Community Projects Foundation, Edinburgh.

Crawford, R. (1977). You are dangerous to your health: the ideology and politics of victim blaming, *Int. J. Hlth Servs.*, **7**, 663–80.

Crawford, R. (1984). A cultural account of 'health': control, release and the social body, in *Issues in the Political Economy of Health Care* (ed, J. B. McKinlay), Tavistock, London, 60–103.

Crozier, M. (1969). *On ne change pas la société par décret*, Grosse-Frasquell, Paris.

Cummins, R. O., Shaper, A. G., Walker, M., and Wale, C. J. (1981). Smoking and drinking by middle-aged British men: effects of social class and town of residence, *BMJ*, **283**, 1497–501.

Cunningham-Burley, S. (1984). The cultural context of childhood illness: unpublished paper presented to British Sociological Association, Medical Sociology Group, Scottish Section.

Curran, J., and Seaton, J. (1985). *Power without Responsibility: The Press and Broadcasting in Britain*, 2nd end, Methuen, London.

Currer, C. (1986). Concepts of mental well and ill-being – the case of Pathan mothers in Britain, in *Concepts of Health, Illness and Disease* (eds. C. Currer and M. Stacey), Berg Publications, Leamington Spa, Hamburg and New York, 183–98.

Currer, C., and Stacey, M. (eds.), (1986). *Concepts of Health, Illness and Disease*, Berg Publications, Leamington Spa, Hamburg, and New York.

Currie, C. E. (1987). Press health coverage in UK national, Scottish national and Scottish local press, Research Unit in Health and Behavioural Change Working Paper, Edinburgh.

Daintree, R. (1986). Medicine and the media, *BMJ*, **293**, 1229.

Dalenius, T. (1977). Bibliography on non-sampling errors in surveys. *Int. Stat. Inst. Rev.*, **49**, 71–90, 181–197, 303–317.

Dalenius, T. (1979). Informed consent or R.S.V.P., in Panel on Incomplete Data of the

Committee on National Statistics/National Research Council, *Symposium on Incomplete Data: Preliminary Proceedings*, US Department of Health, Education and Welfare, Social Security, Washington D.C. Administration, Office of Policy, Office of Research and Statistics, 94–134.

D'Arcy, Masius, Benton & Bowles (1986). *Healthy Eating Study*, D'Arcy, Masius, Benton & Bowles, London.

Davie, R., Butler, N., and Goldstein, H. (1972). *From Birth to Seven*, The Second Report of the National Child Development Study (1958 Cohort), Longman, London.

Davies, J. (1982). The prevention of industrial cancer, in *Prevention of Cancer* (ed. M. Alderson), Edward Arnold, London, 67–78.

Davis, J. A. (1978). Studying categorical data over time, *Soc. Sci. Res.*, **7**, 151–79.

Dayton, S., Pearce, M. L., Hashimoto, S., Dixon, W. J., and Tomiyasu, U. (1969). A controlled clinical trial of a diet high in unsaturated fat in preventing complications of atherosclerosis, *Circulaion*, **40**, Supp. 2, 1–63.

Dean, A., and Lin, N. (1977). The stress-buffering role of social support: problems and prospects for systematic investigation, *J. Nerv. Ment. Dis.*, **165**, 403–17.

Dean, K. (1984). Influence of health beliefs on lifestyles: what do we know? *Eur. Monog. Hlth Ed. Res.*, **6**, 127–49.

Dean, K. (1986). Social support and health: pathways of influence, *Hlth Prom.*, **1**, 133–50.

Derrienic, F. (1977). La mortalité cardiaque des Français actifs d'age moyen selon leur catégorie socio-professionelle et leur région de domicile, *Rev. Epidem. Santé Publ.*, **25**, 131–9.

Detels, R., and Breslow, L. (1984). Current scope, in *Oxford Textbook of Public Health, Volume 1: History, Determinants, Scope, and Strategies* (W. W. Holland, R. Detels and G. Knox, Oxford University Press, Oxford, 20–32.

DHSS (Department of Health and Social Security) (1976. *Prevention and Health: Everybody's Business*, HMSO, London.

DHSS (Department of Health and Social Security) (1977a). *Priorities in the Health Services: The Way Forward*, HMSO, London.

DHSS (Department of Health and Social Security) (1977b). *Prevention and Health*, Cmnd. 7047. HMSO, London.

DHSS (Department of Health and Social Security) (1980). *Inequalities in Health*, report of a Research Working Group, HMSO, London.

DHSS (Department of Health and Social Security) (1984). *Diet and Cardiovascular Disease*, Committee on Medical Aspects of Food Policy, HMSO, London.

DHSS (Department of Health and Social Security) (1986). *Neighbourhood Nursing – A Focus for Care*, report of the Community Nursing Review in England HMSO, London.

Dimsdale, J. E., and Moss, T. (1980). Short-term catecholamine response to psychological stress, *Psychosom. Med.*, **42**, 493–7.

Dingwall, R. (1976). *Aspects of Illness*, Martin Robertson, London.

DOE (Department of the Environment) (1976). *Drinking and Driving*, report of the Departmental Committee, HMSO, London.

Dohrenwend, B. P., and Dohrenwend, B. S. (1969). *Social Status and Psychological Disorder: A Causal Inquiry*, John Wiley & Sons, New York.

Doll, R. (1983). Prospects for prevention, *BMJ*, **286**, 445–8.

Doll, R. Fisher, R. E. W., Gammon, E. H., *et al.* (1965). Mortality of gas workers with special reference to cancer of the lung and bladder, chronic bronchitis and pneumoconiosis, *B. J. Ind. Med.*, **22**, 1–12.

Donovan, J. (1986). *We Don't Buy Sickness. It Just Comes*, Gower, Aldershot, Hants.

Dorkins, H. (1986). The function of the media in the communication of medical information to the public. *The Practitioner*, **230**, 1422 (Suppl.), 1–6.

Douglas, M. (1970). *Natural Symbols: Explorations in Cosmology*, Pantheon, New York.

Draper, P. (1986). Healthy public policy and individual behavioural change: a modern dialectic; unpublished paper (paper presented at the First International Conference on Health Promotion, 17–21 November, Ottawa, Canada).

Draper, P., and Smart, K. (1976). Lessons from the NHS re-organisation, in *Yearbook of Social Policy in Britain 1975* (ed. K. Jones), Routledge and Kegan Paul, London, 37–47.

Draper, P., Best, G., and Dennis, J. (1977). Health and wealth, *Roy. Soc. Hlth, J.*, **97**, 121–6.

Drennan, V. (1985). *Working in a Different Way*, Paddington and North Kensington Health Authority, Health Education Department, London.

Drew, L. (1968). Alcoholism as a self-limiting disease, *Q. J. Stud. Alc.* **29**, 956–66.

Dror, Y. (1964). Muddling through: science or inertia? *Pub. Adm. Rev.*, **24**, 153–7.

Drummond, T. (1975). Using the method of Paulo Freire in nutritional education: an unexperimental plan for community action in northeast Brasil, Carnell International Nutrition, Monograph Series, No. 3.

Dubos, R. (1965). *Man Adapting*, Yale University Press, New Haven, Conn.

Dunnell, K., and Cartwright, A. (1972). *Medicine Takers, Prescribers and Hoarders*, Routledge & Kegan Paul, London.

Durkheim, É. (1897), *Le Suicide*, Paris.

Du Sautoy, P. (1966). Community Development in Britain, *Comm. Dev. J.*, **1**, 1–16.

Earp, J. L., and Ory, M. G. (1978). The effects of social support and health professional home visits on patient adherence to the hypertension regimens; progress report on NIH grant No. HL 18414. (National High Blood Pressure Education Program), Washington D.C.

Eaton, J. W. (1980). Planners as experts in uncertainty? *World Fut. Soc. Bull.*, **March–April**, 27–32.

Eckstein, E. F. (1980). *Food, People and Nutrition*, AVI Publications, Westport.

Egbuonal, R., and Starfield, B. (1982). Child health and social status, *Paediatrics*, 69, 550–7.

Eide, K. (1981). Breaking out of the traditional social policy ghetto, in *The Welfare State in Crisis*, OECD Publications, Paris, 255–60.

Eisenberg, L. (1977). Disease and illness: distinctions between professional and popular ideas of sickness, *Cult. Med. Soc.*, 1, 9–23.

Eklundh, B. L., and Pettersson, B. (1986). *Health Promotion Policy in Sweden – Means and Methods in Intersectorial Action*, National Board of Health and Welfare, Division of Health Education, Stockholm.

Elms, A. (1972). *Social Psychology and Social Relevance*, Little, Brown, Boston, Mass.

Emery, F. (1977). *Futures We Are In*, Martinus Nijhoff Social Services Division. Leiden.

Emrick, C. (1980). A review of psychologically oriented treatment of alcoholism. II: The relative effectiveness of different treatment approaches and the effectiveness of treatment versus no treatment, *J. Stud. Alc.*, **36**, 88–109.

Erikson, E. H. (1959). Identity and the life cycle; selected papers, with a historical introduction by D. Rapapport, *Psychol. Issues*, 1, No. 1 (whole issue).

Etzioni, A. (1967). Mixed-scanning: a third approach to decision making, *Pub. Admin. Rev.*, **27**, 385–92.

Evans-Pritchard, E. E. (1937). *Witchcraft, Oracles and Magic among the Azande*, Clarendon Press, Oxford.

Everitt, B. (1979). Unresolved problems in cluster analysis, *Biometrics*, 35, 169–81.

Fabrega, H. Jr (1971). Medical anthropology, *Bienn. Rev. Anthrop.*, 167–229.

Fabrega, H. Jr (1974). *Disease and Social Behaviour*, MIT Press, Boston, Mass.

Fabrega, H., Jr (1976). Towards a theory of human disease, *J. Nerv. Ment. Dis.*, 162, No. 5, 299–312.

Fabrega, H., Jr., and Manning, P. K. (1979). Illness episodes, illness severity and treatment options in a pluralistic setting, *Soc. Sci. Med.*, 13B, 41–51.

Fagin, L., and Little, M. (1981). *Unemployment and Health in Families*, Department of Health and Social Security, HMSO, London.

Fanning, D. M. (1967). Families in flats, *BMJ*, 4, 382–6.

Farrant, W., and Russell, J. (1986). *The Politics of Health Information*, Bedford Way Paper, 28, University of London, Institute of Education, London.

Featherman, D. L., and Lerner, R. M. (1985). Ontogenesis and sociogenesis: problematics for theory and research about development and socialization across the lifespan, *Am. Soc. Rev.*, **50**, 659–76.

Feinberg, S. E. (1980). *The Analysis of Cross-Classified Categorical Data*, 2nd edn, MIT Press, Cambridge, Mass.

Ferguson, D. M., Horwood, L. J., Shannon, F. T., and Taylor, B. (1981). Parental smoking and former respiratory illness in the first three years of life, *J. Epidem. Comm. Hlth*, 35, 180–4.

Festinger, L. (1957). *A Theory of Cognitive Dissonance*, Row, Peterson, Evanston, Ill.

Feyerabend, P. (1978). *Against Method*, Verso, London.

Fieldhouse, P. (1986). *Food and Nutrition: Customs and Culture*, Croom Helm, London.

Fielding, N. G., and Fielding, J. L. (1986). *Linking Data*, Sage University Paper Series on Qualitative Research Methods, Sage, Beverley Hills, Calif.

Fishbein, M., and Ajzen, I. (1975). *Belief, Attitude, Intention and Behaviour: An Introduction to Theory and Research*, Addison-Wesley, Reading, Mass.

Fisher, S., and Groce, S. B. (1985). Doctor–patient negotiations of cultural assumptions, *Sociol. Hlth Ill.*, **7**, 342–74.

Fitness Systems Inc. (1980). *Corporate Fitness Programs: Trends and Results*, Fitness Systems Inc., Los Angeles, Calif.

Fitzpatrick, R. M. (1982). Social concepts of disease and illness, in *Sociology as Applied to Medicine* (eds. D. L. Patrick and G. Scambler), Balliere's Concise Medical Textbooks, Balliere Tindall, London and Philadelphia, 3–15.

Fletcher, C. (1974). Observations in a surgery, in *Beneath the Surface: An Account of Three Styles of Sociological Research* (ed. C. Fletcher), Routledge & Kegan Paul, London, 71–103.

Fogarty, M. P., and Rapoport, R. (1982). *Families in Britain*, Routledge & Kegan Paul, London.

Foster, G. M. (1975). Medical anthropology: some contrasts with medical sociology, *Soc. Sci. Med.*, **9**, 427–32.

Foucault, M. (1973). *The Birth of the Clinic: An Archaeology of Medical Perception*, Tavistock, London.

Fox, A. J., and Adelstein, A. M. (1978). Occupational mortality: work or way of life? *J. Epiden. Comm. Hlth*, **32**, 73–8.

Fox, A. J., Goldblatt, P. O., and Jones, D. R. (1985). Social class mortality differentials: artefact, selection or life circumstances? *J. Epidem. Comm. Hlth*, **39**, 1–8.

Frankenberg, R. (1980). Medical anthropology and development: a theoretical perspective, *Soc. Sci. Med.*, **14B**, 197–207.

Frankenhaeuser, M. (1975). Experimental approaches to the study of catecholamines and emotions, in *Emotions: Their Parameters and Measurement* (ed. L. Levi), Raven Press, New York, 209–34.

Frazer, W. M. (1950). *A History of Public Health: 1834–1939*, Bailliere, Tindal & Cox, London.

Freidson, E. (1960). Client control and medical practice, *Am. J. Sociol.*, **65**, 374–782.

Freidson, E. (1970a). *Professional Dominance: The Social Structure of Medical Care*, Atherton, New York.

Freidson, E. (1970b). *The Profession of Medicine: A Study of the Sociology of Applied Knowledge*, Dodd Mead, New York.

Freire, P. (1972). *Pedagogy of the Oppressed*, Penguin, Harmondsworth.

Freudenberg, N. (1984–5). Training health educators for social change, *Int. J. Comm. Hlth, Ed.*, **5**, 37–52.

Friedman, G., Spiegelaub, A. B. and Seltzer, C. C. (1973). Cigarette smoking and exposure to occupational hazards. *Am. J. Epidem.*, **98**, 175–83.

Friedmann, J. (1976). *Innovation, Flexibility Response and Social Learning: A Problem in Theory of Meta-Planning*, Geographical Paper, University of Reading.

Fuchs, V. R. (1974). *Who Shall Live?* Basic Books, New York.

Gardner, G., Frank, A. L., and Tuber, L. H. (1984). Effects of social and family factors on viral respiratory infection and illness in the first year of life, *J. Epidem. Comm. Hlth*, **38**, 42–8.

Gardner, M. J., Winter, P. D., and Acheson, E. D. (1982). Variations in cancer mortality among local authority areas in England and Wales: relationship with environmental factors and search for causes, *BMJ*, **284**, 784–7.

Garland, R. (1984). Images of health and medical science conveyed by television, *J. Roy. Coll. Gen. Pract.*, **34**, 316–319.

Gatherer, A., Parfit, J., Porter, E., and Vessey, M. (1979). *Is Health Education Effective? An Overview of Evaluated Studies*, Health Education Council, London.

General Register Office (1987), *Mortality Differentials in Scotland and England and Wales 1969–73 to 1979–83*, General Register Office, Edinburgh.

George, V., and Wilding, P. (1976). *Ideology and Social Welfare*, Routledge & Kegan Paul, London.

Giggs, J. (1986). Ethnic status and mental illness in urban areas, in *Health, Race and Ethnicity* (eds. T. Rathwell and D. Philips), Croom Helm, Kent, 137–74.

Glendon, A. I., and McKenna. S. P. (1985). Using accident injury data to assess the impact of community first aid training, *Pub. Hlth*, **99**, 98–101.

Glick, Z., and Kaufman, N. A. (1976). Weight and skinfold thickness changes during a physical training course, *Med. Sci. Sports*, **8**, 109–12.

Glover, D. (1984). *The Sociology of the Mass Media*, Causeway Press, Ormskirk, Lancs., England.

Goffman, E. (1963). *Behaviour in Public Places*, Free Press, Glencoe, New York.

Goldberg, D. P., and Huxley, P. (1982). *Mental Illness in the Community*, Tavistock, London.

Goldberg, S. M., and Morrison, S. (1963). 'Schizophrenia and Social Class', *B. J. Psychiat.*, **109**, 785–91.

Goldthorpe, J. H. (1980). *Social Mobility and Class Structures in Modern Britain*, Clarendon Press, Oxford.

Goodman, L. A. (1973). Causal analysis of data from panel studies and other kinds of surveys, *Am. J. Sociol.*, **78**, 1135–91.

Goodman, L. A. (1979). A brief guide to the causal analysis of data from surveys, *Am. J. Sociol.*, **84**, 1078–95.

Goodman, L. A. (1984). *The Analysis of Cross-classified Date Having Ordered Categories*, Harvard University Press, Cambridge, Mass.

Graham, H. (1982). Coping: or how mothers are seen and not heard, in *On the Problem of Men* (eds. S. Friedman and E. Sarah), Women's Press, London, 101–16.

Graham, H. (1984). *Women, Health and the Family*, Wheatsheaf Books, Harvester, Sussex.

Graham, H. (1986). Women smoking and family health; paper presented at British Sociological Association Medical Sociology Group Conference, September, York.

Graham, H., and Oakley, A. (1981). Competing ideologies of reproduction: medical and maternal perspectives on pregnancy and childbirth, in *Women, Health and Reproduction*, (ed. H. Roberts), Routledge & Kegan Paul, London, 50–74.

Green, L. (1984). Health education models, in *Behavioural Health: A Handbook of Health Enhancement and Disease Prevention* (eds). J. Matarazzo. S. Weiss, J. Herd. and N. Miller), John Wiley, New York, 181–98.

Green, L. W. Kreuter, M., Deeds, S., and Partridge, K. (1980). *Health Education Planning: A Diagnostic Approach*, Mayfield Press, Palo Alto, Calif.

Grind, J. (ed.) (1982). *Helseplan for 1980 Aara*, Gyldendal Norsk Forlag, Oslo.

Gruchow, W. (1979). Catecholamine activity and infectious disease episodes, *J. Hum. Stress*, **5**, 11–17.

Gusfield, J. (1975). Categories of ownership and responsibility in social issues: alcohol abuse and automobile use, *J. Drug Issues*, **5**, 290–5.

Gustavesen, B. (1986). Social research as participative dialogue, in *The Use and Abuse of Social Science* (ed. F. Heller), Sage, London, 143–56.

Gyr Brown, J. S., Willey, R., and Zivian, A. (1966). Computer simulation and psychological theories of perception, *Psychol. Bull.*, **65**, 174–92.

Haggerty, R. J. (1977). Changing lifestyles to improve health, *Prev. Med.* **6**, 276–89.

Hall, M. H., Chng, P. K., and MacGillvray, I. (1980). Is routine antenatal care worthwhile?, *Lancet*, **ii**, 78–80.

Hallett, R., and Sutton, S. (1986). Factors influencing the decision to attempt to stop smoking in a media-based smoking intervention programme, *Hlth Ed. Res.*, **1**, 163–73.

Halsey, A. H. (1981). *Changes in British Society*, Tavistock, London.

Hammond, E. C., and Selikoff, I. J. (1975). Multiple risk factors in environmental cancer, in *Persons at High Risk of Cancer* (ed. J. Fraumeni), Academic Press, New York.

Hancock, T. (1960). The soft path: no alternative future for health in the 1980's, in *Through the 80's: Thinking Global: Acting Locally* (ed. World Future Society), World Future Society Publications, Washington, 352–5.

Hancock, T. (1982). The soft health path: a healthier future for physicians?, *J. Can. Med. Ass.*, **126**, 1019–20.

Hancock, T. (1985). Beyond health care: from Public health policy to healthy public policy, *Can. J. Pub. Hlth*, **76**, (Supplement 1), 9–11.

Hancock, T. (1986). Lalonde and beyond: looking back at a new perspective on the health of Canadians, *Hlth Prom.*, **1**, 93–100.

Hancock, T. C., and Perkins, F. (1985), The Mandala of Health: a conceptual model and teaching tool, *Hlth Ed.*, **24**, 8–10.

Hannay, D. R. (1979). *The Symptom Iceberg: A Study of Community Health*, Routledge & Kegan Paul, London.

Hanson, J. S., Tabakin, B. S., Levy, A. M., and Nedde, W. (1968). Long-term physical training and cardiovascular dynamics in middle-aged men, *Circulation*, **38**, 783–99.

Harkey, J., Miles, D. L., and Rushing, W. A. (1976). The relationship between social class and functional status: a new look at the drift hypothesis, *J. Hlth, Soc. Behav.*, **17**, 194–204.

Harper, A. L. (1983). Coronary heart disease – an epidemic related to diet? *Am. J. Clin. Nutr.*, **37**, 669–81.

Harris, D. M., and Guten, S. (1979). Health protective behaviour: an exploratory study, *J. Hlth Soc. Behav.*, **20**, 17–29.

Hartley, E. L. (ed). (1947). *Readings in Social Psychology*, Holt, Rinehart & Winston, New York, 197–211.

Hartley, J. F. (1980). The impact of unemployment upon the self-esteem of managers, *J. Occup. Psychol.*, **53**, 147–55.

Harwood, A. (1971). The hot–cold theory of disease. Implications for treatment of Puerto Rican patients, *J. Am. Med. Ass.*, **216**, 1153–68.

Havighurst, R. (1952). *Developmental Tasks and Education*, Longmans Green, New York.

Haynes, D., and Ross, C. E. (1986). Body and mind: the effect of exercise overnight, and physical health on psychological well-being, *J. Hlth Soc., Behav.*, **27**, 387–400.

Haynes, S. G., Feinleib, M., and Kannell, B. (1980). The relationship of psychosocial factors to coronary heart disease in the Framingham Study: III, Eight-year incidence of coronary heart disease, *Am. J. Epidem.*, **III**, 37–58.

Heasman, M., and Lipworth, L. (1969). *Accuracy of Certification of Cause of Death*, HMSO, London.

Heather, N., Roberton, I., and Davies, P. (1985). *The Misuse of Alcohol*, Croom Helm, London.

Heclo, H. (1972). Policy analysis, *B. J. Pol. Sci.*, **2**, 83–108.

Heinzelmann, F., and Bagley, R. W. (1970). Responses to physical activity programmes and their effects on health behaviour *Pub. Hlth Reps.*, **85**, 905–11.

Heller, F. (ed.) (1986). *The Use and Abuse of Social Science*, Sage, London.

Helman, C. G. (1978). 'Feed a cold, starve a fever'. Folk models of infection in an English suburban community and their relation to medical treatment, *Cult. Med. Soc.*, **2**, 107–37.

Helsing, E. (1986). The Norwegian nutrition policy: research programme on measures for its implementation; report on a seminar in Sanner, Norway, 16–17 January, WHO, Copenhagen.

Henderson, S., Byrne, D., Duncan-Jones, P., Adcock, S., Scott, S., and Steele, G. (1978). Social bands in the epidemiology of neurosis: a preliminary investigation, *B. J. Psychiat.*, **32**, 463–6.

Hennekens, C. H., Rosner, B., and Cole, D. S. (1978). Daily alcohol consumption and fatal coronary heart disease, *Am. J. Epidem.*, **107**, 196–200.

Henry, J. P. (1982). The relation of social to biological processes in disease, *Soc. Sci. Med.*, **16**, 369–80.

Henry, J. P., and Stephens, P. M. (1977). *Stress, Health and the Social Environment: A Sociobiological Approach to Medicine*, Springer-Verlag New York.

Hepworth, S. J. (1980). Moderating factors of the psychological impact of unemployment, *J. Occup. Psychol.*, **53**, 139–45.

Herman, C. P., and Mack, D. (1975). Restricted and unrestricted eating. *J. Pers.*, **43**, 647–60.

Herzlich, C. (1973). *Health and Illness*, Academic Press, London.

Herzlich, C., and Pierret, J. (1986). Illness: from causes to meaning, in *Concepts of Health, Illness and Disease* (eds. C. Currer and M. Stacey), Berg Publications, Leamington Spa, Hamburg and New York, 73–96.

HMSO (Her Majesty's Stationery Office) (1944). *A National Health Service*, Coalition Government White Paper. Cmnd. 6502 HMSO, London.

Hogwood, B. W., and Gunn, L. A. (1984). *Policy Analysis for the Real World*, Oxford University Press, Oxford.

Holland, S. (1979). The development of an action and counselling service in a deprived urban area, in *New Methods of Mental Health Care* (ed. M. Meacher), Pergamon, Oxford, 95–106.

Hollingshead, A. B. (1965). *Two Factor Index of Social Position* (privately printed). Yale Station, New Haven, Conn.

Holmes, T. H., and Masua, M. (1974). Life change and illness susceptibility, in *Stressful Life Events: Their Nature and Effects* (eds. B. S. Dohrenwend and B. P. Dohrenwend), John Wiley & Sons, New York, 45–76.

Holmes, T. H., and Rahe, R. H. (1967). The social readjustment rating scale, *J. Psychosom. Res.*, 11, 213–18.

Holterman, S. (1975). Areas of urban deprivation in Great Britain. An analysis of 1971 Census data, *Social Trends*, No. 6, 33038, HMSO, London.

Homans, G. C. (1961). *Social Behaviour: Its Elementary Forms*, Harcourt, Brace and World Inc. New York.

Horn, D. (1968). Factors affecting the cessation of cigarette smoking: a prospective study: paper presented at the Meeting of the Eastern Psychological Association, Washington DC.

Horn, D. (1972). Determinants of change, in *The 2nd World Conference on Smoking and Health* (ed. G. Richardson), Pitman Medical Press, London, 9–18.

Horne, D. J. de L., and McCormack, H. (1984). Behavioural psychotherapy for a blood and needle phobia mastectomy patient receiving adjuvant chemotherapy, *Behav. Psychother.*, 12, 342–8.

Hosen, H. (1978). Moulds in allergy, *J. Asthma Res.*, 15, 151–6.

House, J. S., Robbins, C., Metzner, H. L., *et al.* (1982). The association of social relationships and activities with mortality: prospective evidence from the Tecumsheh community health study, *Am. J. Epidem.*, 116, 123–40.

d'Houtaud, A., and Field, M. G. (1984). The image of health: variations in perception by social class in a French population, *Sociol. Hlth, Ill.*, 6, 30–60.

d'Houtaud, A., and Field, M. G. (1986). New research on the image of health, in *Concepts of Health, Illness and Disease* (eds C. Currer and M. Stacey), Berg Publications, Leamington Spa, Hamburg, and New York, 235–55.

Hovland, C. I., Lumsdaine, A. A., and Sheffield, F. D. (1949). *Experiments on Mass Communication*, Princeton University Press, Princeton, N.J.

Huckfeldt, R. R., Kohfeld, C. W., and Likens, T. W. (1982). *Dynamic Modeling: An Introduction*, Sage Publications, Beverly Hills.

Hull, D. (1976). Life circumstances and physical illness: a cross-disciplinary survey of research content and method for the decade 1965–1975. *J. Psychosom. Res.*, 21, 115–19.

Hunt, R. N. (1977). *Peace River FACTS Project: Final Statistical Report*, Grande Prairie Regional College, Alberta.

Hunt, S. (1985). Below the breadline, *Community Outlook*, **October**, 19–21.

Hunt, S. M. (1984. Health indicators and social deprivation in Camberwell: report to Camberwell Health Authority, London.

Hunt, S. M. (1987). Subjective health indicators for health promotion research, Research Unit in Health and Behavioural Change Working Paper, Edinburgh.

Hunt, S. M., Currie, C., and Martin, C. J. (1987). Food and fibre in a Scottish community, *Hlth Ed. Res.*, 3, 223–9.

Hunt, S. M., McEwen, J., and McKenna, S. P. (1985). Social inequalities and perceived health, *Effective Health Care*, 2, 151–60.

Hunt, S. M., and MacLeod, M. (1987). Health and behavioural change: some lay perspectives, *Comm. Med.*, 9, 68–76.

Hunt, S. M. and Martin, C. J. (1988). Health-related behavioural change: A test of a new model. *Psych. & Hlth.*, in press.

Hunt, S. M., Morrison, M., and Jones, J. (1986). Prescribing patterns in an Edinburgh group practice; unpublished paper, Research Unit in Health and Behavioural Change, Edinburgh.

Hunt, W. A., and Matarazzo, J. D. (1970). Habit mechanisms in smoking, in *Learning Mechanisms in Smoking* (ed. W. Hunt), Aldive, Chicago, 65–90.

Hunt, W. A., Matarazzo, J. D., Weiss, S. M., and Gentry, W. D. (1967). Associative learning, habit and health behaviour, *J. Behav. Med.*, 2, 111–24.

Hunter, D. (1975). *The Diseases of Occupations*, 5th ed, English University Press, London.

Hunter, D. (1987). Any which way but loose: the challenge of joint planning, *Link Up*, ECSS, April 1987.

Hunter, D. J. (1980). *Coping with Uncertainty: Policy and Politics in the National Health Service*, Research Study Press, Chichester.

Idler, E. L. (1979). Definitions of health and illness in medical sociology, *Soc. Sci. Med.*, **13A**, 723–31.

Illich, I. (1975). *Medical Nemesis*, Calder & Boyars, London.

Illsley, R. (1955). Social class, selection and class differences in relation to still births and infant deaths, *BMJ*, **ii**, 1590.

Illsely, R. (1967). Sociological study of reproduction and its outcome, in *Childbirth in its Social and Psychological Aspects* (eds S. A. Richardson and A. F. Guttmacher), Williams & Wilkins, New York, 75–141.

Illsley, R. (1980). *Professional or Public Health?* Rock Carling Fellowship 1980, Nuffield Provincial Hospitals Trust, London.

Illsley, R. (1986). Occupational class, selection and the production of inequalities, *Quart. J. Soc. Aff.*, **2**, 151–65.

Illsley, R., and Mullen, K. (1985). The health needs of disadvantaged client groups, in *Oxford Textbooks of Public Health, Volume 4: Specific Applications* (eds, W. W. Holland, R. Detels and G. Knox), Oxford University Press, Oxford, 389–402.

Jacobson, B. (1981). *The Lady Killers: Why Smoking is a Feminist Issue*, Pluto Press, London.

Jaeckel, M. (1971). Coleman's process approach, in *Sociological Methodology: 1971* (ed. H. L. Costner), Jossey-Bass, San Francisco.

James, W. (1891). *The Principles of Psychology, Volume 1*, Macmillan, London.

Janis, I., and Mano, L. (1965). Effectiveness of emotional role playing on the desire to modify smoking habits and attitudes, *J. Exp. Res. Pers.*, **7**, 17–27.

Janis, I. L., and Field, P. B. (1956). A behavioural assessment of persuasibility: consistency of individual differences, *Sociometry*, **19**, 241–53.

Jemmott, J. B., III, and Locke, S. E. (1984). Psychosocial factors, immunilogic mediation and human susceptibility to infectious disease: how much do we know? *Psychol. Bull.*, **95**, 78–108.

Jenkins, J. (1983). Women poorly advised by Channel 4, *BMJ*, **286**, 802–3.

JICNARS (Joint Industry Committee for National Readership Surveys) (1984). *National Readership Survey 1984*, JICNARS, London.

Jensen, M. A. (1987). Understanding addictive behaviour: implications for health promotion programming, *Am. J. Hlth Prom.*, **1**, 48–57.

John Hopkins School of Hygiene and Public Health (1982). *Circular: 1982–83*, John Hopkins University, Baltimore, Md.

Johnson, J. V. (1986). *The Impact of Workplace Social Support, Job Demand and Work Control upon Cardiovascular Disease in Sweden*, Report No. 1, Department of Psychology, University of Stockholm.

Johnson, R. (1976), *The Ethical Aspects of Government Intervention into Individual Behaviour*, Staff Papers, Long Range Health Planning, Department of National Health and Welfare, Canada, Ottawa.

Joint Industry Committee for National Readership Surveys (1984). *National Readership Survey*; 1985, Jicnars, London.

Jones, I. G., and Cameron, D. (1984). Social class analysis: an embarrassment to epidemiology, *Comm. Med.*, **6**, 37–46.

Jones, J. (1983). *Community Development and Health Issues*, Community Projects Foundation, Edinburgh.

Joreskog, K., and Sorbom, D. (1982). *LISREL V: Analysis of Linear Structural Relationships by the Method of Maximum Likelihood*, International Educational Services, Chicago.

Kandel, D. B., Davies, M., and Raveis, V. H. (1985). The stressfulness of daily social roles for women: marital, occupational and household roles, *J. Hlth Soc. Behav.*, **26**, 64–78.

Kangesu, E. (1984). *Springfield Hospital Admission Survey*, Camberwell Health Authority, London.

Kaplan, B. H., *et al.* (1983). The epidemiological evidence for a relationship between social support and health, *Am. J. Epidem.*, **117**, 521–37.

Kaptein, A. A. (1984). *Illness Behaviour of Patients with Asthma*, Vrije Universiteit te Amsterdam, Amsterdam.

Karapin, R. S. (1986). What's the use of social science? A review of the literature, in *The Use and Abuse of Social Science* (ed. F. Heller), Sage, London, 236–65.

Karasek, R., Baker, D., Marxer, F., Ahlbom, A., and Theorell, T. (1981). Job decision, job demands and cardio-vascular disease: a prospective study of Swedish men, *A. J. Pub Hlth*, **71**, 695–705.

Kasl, S., Cobb, S., and Brooks, G. W. (1975). The experience of losing a job: reported changes in health, symptoms and illness behaviour, *Psychosom. Med.*, **10**, 3–10.

Kasl, S. V., and Cooper, C. L. (1987). *Stress and Health: Issues in Research Methodology*, John Wiley and Sons, Chichester.

Keehn, R. J. (1974). Probability of death related to previous army rank. *Lancet*, **20**, 170–2.

Kelly, G. (1955). *The Psychology of Personal Constructs, Volume 1. A Theory of Personality*, Norton, New York.

Kelman, H. C. (1969). Processes of opinion change, in *The Planning of Change: Readings in the Applied Behavioural Sciences* (eds. W. Bennes, K. Bennes and R. Chin), Holt, Rinehart & Winston, New York, 131–58.

Kelman, S. (1975). The social nature of the definition problem in health, *Int. J. Hlth Servs.*, **5**, 609–38.

Kemeny, J. G. (1952). *A Philosopher Looks at Science*, D. Van Nostrand, Princeton, NJ.

Kennedy, I. (1980). Showbiz and the doctors – why Panorama was wrong, *Sunday Times*, **30** November, 16.

Kerr, M., and Charles, N. (1986). Servers and providers: the distribution of food within the family, *Sociol. Rev.*, **34**, 115–57.

Kessler, R. C., and Greenberg, D. F. (1981). *Linear Panel Analysis: Models of Quantitative Change*, Academic Press, New York.

Key, M., Hudson, P., and Armstrong, J. (1985). *Evaluation Theory and Community Work*, Community Projects Foundation, London.

Kickbush, I. (1986a). Health promotion: a global perspective, Keynote Address to the 77th Canadian Public Health Association Annual Conference in 16–19 June, Vancouver, Canada.

Kickbush, I. (1986b). Life-styles and health, *Soc. Sci. Med.*, **22**, 117–24.

Kiesler, C. A., and Kiesler, S. B. (1969). *Conformity*, Addison-Wesley, Reading, Mass.

King, N. J., and Remenyi, A. (1986). *Health Care: A Behavioural Approach*, Grune & Stratton, New York.

Kirsht, J. P. (1974). The health belief model and illness behaviour, *Hlth Ed. Monog.*, **2**, 287–408.

Kirsht, J. P., and Rosenstock, I. M. (1977). Patient adherence to antihypertensive medical regimens, *J. Comm. Hlth*, **3**, 115–19.

Kitsuse, J., and Spector, M. (1975). Social problems and deviance: some parallel issues, *Soc. Probs.*, **22**, 584–94.

Kleinman, A. (1978). Concepts and a model for the comparison of medical systems as cultural systems, *Soc. Sci. Med.*, **12**, 85–93.

Knapper, C., and Warr, P. B. (1965). The effect of position and layout on the readership of news items, *Gazette* II, 323–8.

Knoke, D., and Burke, P. J. (1980). *Log–Linear Models*, Sage Publications, Beverley Hills.

Koskinen, S. (1985). Time trends in cause specific mortality by occupational class in England and Wales; paper presented at the IUSSP 20th General Conference, Florence.

Kreitman, N., and Platt, S. (1984). Suicide, unemployment and domestic gas detoxification in Britain, *J. Epidem. Comm. Hlth.*, **38**, 1–6.

Kiristiansen, C. M. (1983). Newspaper coverage of diseases and actual mortality statistics, *Eur. J. Soc. Psychol.*, **13**, 193–4.

Kristiansen, C. M., and Harding, C. M. (1984). Mobilization of health behavior by the press in Britain, *Journalism Quart.*, **61**, 364–70.

Kristiansen, C. M., and Harding, C. M. (1988). A comparison of the coverage of health issues by Britain's quality and popular press, *Hlth Ed. Res.*, (In Press).

Kuo, W. H., and Yung-Mei, T. (1986). Social networking, hardiness and immigrant's mental health, *J. Hlth Soc. Behav.*, **27**, 133–49.

Kurland, A., (1978). *Psychiatric Aspects of Opiate Dependence*, CRC Press, West Palm Beach, Fla.

Kuter, B., Wilkins, C., and Yarrow, P. R. (1952). Verbal attitudes and overt behaviour involving racial prejudice, *J. Abn. Soc. Psychol.*, **47**, 649–55.

Labonte, R. (1986). Social inequalities and healthy public policy, in *Hlth Prom.*, **1**, 341–52.

Labonte, R., and Penfold, S. (1981). Canadian perspectives in health promotion, *Hlth Ed.*, **19**, 4–7.

Labovitz, S. (1972). Statistical usage in sociology: sacred cows and ritual, *Sociol. Meth. Res.*, **1**, 13–37.

Lacey, J., Pepys, J., and Cross, T. (1972). Actinomycetes and fungus spores in air as respiratory allergens, in *Safety in Microbiology* (eds, D. A. Shapton and R. G. Board), Academic Press, London, 45–64.

Lajer, M. (1982). Unemployment and hospitalisation among bricklayers, *Scand. J. Soc. Med.*, **10**, 3–10.

Lalonde, M. (1974). *A New Perspective on the Health of Canadians – A Working Document*, Minister of Health and Welfare, Ottawa.

Land, K. C. (1969). Principles of path analysis, in *Sociological Methodology: 1969* (ed. E. Borgatta), Jossey-Bass, San Francisco, 3–37.

Land, K. C. (1976). A general framework for building dynamic macro social indicator models: including an analysis of changes in crime rates and police expenditures, *Am. J. Sociol.*, **82**, 565–604.

Lang, T. (1984). *Jam Tomorrow?* Food Policy Unit, Manchester Polytechnic, Manchester.

La Pierre, R. T. (1934). Attitudes versus actions, *Social Forces*, **13**, 238–7.

Lauzon, R. R. J. (1977). A randomised controlled trial of the application of Health Hazard Appraisal to stimulus approach risk reduction behaviour, *Proceedings of the 13th Meeting of the Society for Prospective Medicine*, 102–3.

Lawrence, P. S. (1958). Chronic illness and socio-economic status, in *Patients, Physicians and Illness*, (ed. E. Gartly Jaco), Free Press, Glencoe, New York, 37–49.

Lazarus, A. (1971). *Behaviour Therapy and Beyond*, McGraw-Hill, New York.

LCHR (London Community Health Resource) (1986). *Measuring Change, Making Changes – An Approach to Evaluation*, LCHR, London.

Lefebvre, R., Peterson, G., McGraw, S., Lasater, T., Sennett, L., Kendall, L., and Carleton, R. (1986). Community intervention to lower blood cholesterol in the 'know your cholesterol' campaign in Pawtucket, Rhode Island, *Hlth Ed. Quart.*, **13**, 117–29.

Leon, A. S., Conrad, J., Hunninghake, D. D., and Serfass, R. (1979). Effects of a vigorous walking programme on body composition and carbohydrate and lipid metabolism of obese young men, *Am. J. Nutr.*, **32**, 1776–87.

Leon, G. (1976). Current directions in the treatment of obesity, *Psychol Bull*, **83**, 557–78.

Lessler, J. R. (1979). An expanded survey error model, In *Symposium on Incomplete Data: Preliminary Proceedings*, US Department of Health Education and Welfare, Washington D.C. 55–63.

Letourmy, A. (1986). Qui veut en France d'un mode de vie plus sain?, *Soc. Sci. Med.*, **22**, 125–133.

Leventhal, H., and Cleary, P. (1980). The smoking problem: a review of the research and theory in behavioural risk modification, *Psychol. Bull.*, **88**, 370–405.

Leventhal, H., Watts, J. C., and Pagano, F. (1967). Effects of fear and instructions on how to cope with danger, *J. Pers. Soc. Psychol.*, **6**, 313–19.

Levin, L. S., Katz, A. H., and Holst, E. (1977). *Self Care: Lay Initiatives in Health*, Croom Helm, London.

Lewin, K, (1947). Group decision and social change, in *Readings in Social Psychology* (eds. E. E. Maccoby, T. M. Newcomb and E. L. Hartley), Holt, Rinehart & Winston, New York, 197–211.

Lewis, J. (1986). *What Price Community Medicine: The Philosophy, Practice, and Politics of Public Health since 1919*, Wheatsheaf, Brighton, Sussex.

Lewis, S., Haskell, W. L., Wood, P. D., Manoogian, N., Bailey, J. E., and Pereiva, M. (1976). Effects of physical activity on weight reduction in obese middle-aged women, *Am. J. Clin. Nutr.*, **29**, 151–6.

Ley, P. (1977). Psychological and behavioural factors in weight loss, in *Recent Advances in Obesity*

Research II (ed. G. Bray), Proceedings of the Second International Congress on Obesity, Washington DC, Newman, London.

Lichstenstein, E. (1982). The smoking problem: a behavioural perspective, *J. Consult, Clin. Psychol.*, **50**, 804–19.

Lieban, R. W. (1974). Medical anthropology, in *Handbook of Social and Cultural Anthropology* (ed. J. J. Honigman), Rand McNally, Chicago, 1031–72.

Lieberman, M. A. (1961). Relationship of mortality rates to entrance to a home for the aged, *Geriatrics*, **16**, 515–19.

Light, R. J., and Smith, P. V. (1970). Choosing future strategies for designing and evaluating new programs, *Harvard Ed. Rev.*, **40**, 1–28.

Lindley, D. V., and Smith, A. F. M. (1972). Bayes estimates for the linear model [with discussion], *J. Roy. Stat. Soc.*, **Series B 34**, 1–41.

Lock, S. (1986). Medicine and the media, *BMJ*, **293**, 1228–9.

Locker, D. (1981). *Symptoms and Illness: the Cognitive Organisation of Disorder*, Tavistock, London.

Love, R., and Kalnis, I. (1984). Individualist and structuralist perspectives on nutrition education for Canadian children, *Soc. Sci. Med.*, **18**, 199–205.

Lovejoy, A. O. (1948). *Essays in the History of Ideas*, Johns Hopkins Press, Baltimore, Md.

Lundin, F. E., Wagoner, J. K., and Archer, V. E. (1971). *Radon Daughter Exposure and Respiratory Cancer, Quantitative and Temporal Aspects*, National Institute of Occupational Safety and Health and National Institute, Environmental Health and Safety, Joint Monograph No. 1, USDHEW, Washingston DC.

Luria, A. (1973), *The Working Brain*, Allen Lane, Penguin, Harmondsworth, Middx.

Luria, A. R., Simernitskaya, E. G., and Tubylevich, B. (1970). The structure of psychological processes in relation to cerebral organisation, *Neuropsych.*, **8**, 217–31.

Mackintosh, J. M. (1953). *Trends of Opinion about the Public Health: 1901–51*, Oxford University Press, London.

Maclean, P. D. (1959). The limbic system in respect to two basic life principles, in *The CNS and Behaviour: Transactions of the Second Conference of the Josiah Macy Jr. Foundation* (ed. M. Brazier), New York, 106–32.

MacMahon, B., and Pugh, T. F. (1970). *Epidemiology: Principles and Methods*, Little, Brown, Boston, Mass.

McCloskey, H. E. (1965). A critique of ideals of liberty, *Mind*, **74**, 483–508.

McCombs, M. E., and Shaw, D. L. (1972). The agenda setting function of the mass media, *Publ. Opin. Quart.*, **36**, 176–87.

McFall, R. (1978). Smoking cessation research, *J. Consult. Clin. Psych.*, **46**, 703–12.

McFall, R. M. (1970). The effect of self-monitoring of normal smoking behaviour, *J. Consult. Clin. Psychol.*, **35**, 135–42.

McGill, A. M. (1978). A national high blood pressure education research program. Abstracts of papers presented at the 1st International Congress on Patient Counselling, *Pat. Couns. Hlth Ed.*, **1**, 35.

McKee, I. (1984). Community antenatal care: the Sighthill Community Antenatal Scheme, in *Pregnancy Care for the 1980's* (eds. L. Zarder and G. Chamberlain), RSM/MacMillan, London, 32–41.

McKenna, S. P., and Hale, A. R. (1982). Changing behaviour towards danger: the effect of first aid training, *J. Occup. Accid.*, **4**, 47–50.

McKeown, T. (1965). *Medicine in Modern Society*, Routledge & Kegan Paul, London.

McKeown, T. (1976). *The Role of Medicine: Dream, Mirage or Nemesis*, Nuffield Provincial Hospitals Trust, London.

McKeown, T. (1980). *The Role of Medicine: Dream, Mirage or Nemesis*, 2nd Edn, Basil Blackwell, Oxford.

McKinlay, J. B. (1975). The help seeking behaviour of the poor, in *Poverty and Health*, (eds. J. Kosa and I. K. Zoca), Harvard University Press, Cambridge, Mass, 224–73.

McMillan, J. S. (1957). Examination of the association between housing conditions and pulmonary T. B. in Glasgow, *B. J. Prev. Soc. Med.*, **11**, 142–51.

McMorrow, M. J., and Fox, R. M. (1983). Nicotine's role in smoking: an analysis of nicotine regulation, *Psychol. Bull.*, **93**, 102–27.

McQuail, D. (1976). Review of sociological writing on the press, Royal Commission Press Working Paper, No. 2, HMSO, London.

McQueen, D. V. (1985). The Women's Health Shop in Edinburgh, Research Unit in Health and Behavioural Change Working Paper No. 2, Edinburgh.

McQueen, D. V. (1986a). Directions for research in health behaviour related to health promotion: a general overview, Research Unit in Health and Behavioural Change Working Paper No. 6, Edinburgh

McQueen, D. V. (1986b). Health education research: the problem of linkages, *Hlth Ed. Res.*, **1**, 289–94.

McQueen, D. V. (1987a). Telephone interviewing and CATI, Research Unit in Health and Behavioural Change Working Paper No. 1, Edinburgh.

McQueen, D. V. (1987b). A research programme in lifestyle and health: methodological and theoretical considerations, *Rev. Epidem. Santé Pub.*, **35**, 28–35.

McQueen, D. V. (1987c). Sampling issues, Research Unit in Health and Behavioural Change Working Paper No. 3, Edinburgh.

McQueen, D. V., and Celentano, D. D. (1982). Social factors in the etiology of multiple outcomes, *Soc. Sci. Med.*, **16**, 397–418.

McQueen, D. V., and Siegrist, J. (1982). Social factors in the etiology of chronic disease: an overview, *Soc. Sci. Med.*, **16**, 353–67.

Madeley, R. (1978). Relating child health services to needs by the use of simple epidemiology, *Pub. Hlth*, **92**, 224–38.

Mahler, H. (1986). Address to the First International Conference on Health Promotion, *Hlth Prom.*, **1**, 409–12.

Mahoney, M. J., and Mahoney, K. (1976). *Permanent Weight Control*, Norton, New York.

Manning, P. K., and Fabrega, H., Jr (1973). The experience of self and body: health and illness in the Chiapas Highlands, in *Phenomenological Sociology* (ed. G. Psathas), John Wiley & Sons, New York, 251–301.

Maris, R. (1970). The logical adequacy of Homans' social theory, *Am. Sociol. Rev.*, **35**, 1069–81.

Marmot, M. G., Booth, M., and Beral, V. (1981). Changes in heart disease mortality in England and Wales, *Hlth Trends*, **13**, 33–8.

Marmot, M. G., and Madge, N. (1987). An epidemiological perspective on stress and health, in *Stress and Health: Issues in Research Methodology* (eds. S. V. Kasl and C. L. Cooper), John Wiley & Sons, Chichester, Sussex 3–26.

Marsh, A. (1985). Smoking and illness: what smokers really believe. *Hlth Trends*, **17**, 7–12.

Martin, C. J., Brown, G. W., and Brockington, I. F. (1982). Psycho-social stress and puerperal psychiatric disorder; paper presented at Marce Society Conference, London.

Martin, C. J., Platt, S. D., and Hunt, S. M. (1987). Housing conditions and ill health, *BMJ*, **294**, 1125–7.

Martin, F. M. (1977). Social medicine and its contribution to social policy, *Lancet*, **24 December** 1336–8.

Martin, F. M., Brotherston, J. H. F., and Chave, S. P. W. (1957). The incidence of neurosis in a new housing estate, *B. J. Prev. Soc. Med.*, **11**, 196–202.

Masini, E. (1982). Reconceptualization futures: a need and a hope, *World Fut. Soc. Bull.*, **November-December**, 1–8.

Mason, W. M., Wong, G. Y., and Entwistle, B. (1983). Contextual analysis through the multilevel linear model, in *Sociological Methodology: 1983-1984* (ed. S. Leinhardt), Jossey-Bass, London, 72–103.

Matarazzo, J. D., Weiss, S. M., and Herd, J. A. (1984). *Behavioural Health: A Handbook of Health Enhancement and Disease Prevention*, John Wiley & Sons, New York.

Maunsell, K. (1954). Sensitisation risk from inhalation of fungal spores, *J. Laryngol. Otol.*, **68**, 765–75.

Mead, G. H. (1934). *Mind, Self and Society*, University of Chicago Press, Chicago.

Meadows, S. H. (1963). Social class migration and chronic bronchitis, *B. J. Soc. Med.*, **15**, 171–5.

Mechanic, D. (1968). *Medical Sociology*, Free Press, New York.

Medical News (1983). Nurses and smoking, *BMJ*, **286**, 233.

Milgram, S. (1974). *Obedience to Authority*, Tavistock, London.

Milio, N. (1976). A framework for prevention: changing health-damaging to health-generating life patterns, *Am. J. of Pub. Hlth*, **64**, 435–8.

Milio, N. (1977). An ecological approach to health planning for illness prevention, *Am. J. of Publ. Hlth*, **67**, 7–10.

Milio, N. (1981). Promoting health through structural change: analysis of the origins and implementation of Norway's farm-food-nutrition policy, *Soc. Sci. Med.*, **15A**, 721–34.

Milio, N. (1983). *Promoting Health Through Public Policy*, F. A. Davis, Philadelphia, Pa.

Millar, P. Mc. C., and Ingham, J. (1976). Friends, confidants and symptoms, *Soc. Psychiat.*, **11**, 51–8.

Miller, E., and Edwards, J. (1982). The unequal society: a challenge to public health; report to the City of Toronto, Department of Public Health and Planning and Department of Development.

Miller, G., and Agnew, N., (1973). First aid training and accidents, *Occup. Psychol.*, **47**, 209.

Miller, G., Galanter, E., and Pribram, K. (1965). *Plans and the Structure of Behaviour*, Holt, Rinehart & Winston, New York.

Miller, P. V., and Cannell, C. F. (1982). A study of experimental techniques for telephone interviewing, *Pub. Op. Quart.*, **46**, 250–69.

Miller, W. R. (ed). (1980). *The Addictive Behaviours*, Pergamon, Oxford.

Mills, J. S. (1909), *Principles of Political Economy*, Longmans, London.

Milsum, J. H., Laszlo, C. A., and Prince, P. R. (1976). A pilot evaluation of introducing Health Hazard Appraisal in a community health centre environment, *Proceedings of the 12th Meeting of the Society of Prospective Medicine*, 92–102.

Ministry of Agriculture, Fisheries and Food (1976). *Household Food Consumption and Expenditure*, National Food Survey, London.

Ministry of Health and General Register Office (1967). *Reports of Hospital Inpatient Enquiry for the Two Years 1960 and 1961*, part III, HMSO, London.

Mitchell, J. R. A. (1985). Diet and cardiovascular disease – the myths and the realities, *Proc. Nutr. Soc.*, **44**, 363–70.

Mitchell, R. E., and Moos, R. H. (1984). Deficiencies in social support among depressed patients: antecedents or consequences of stress, *J. Hlth Soc, Behav.*, **25**, 438–52.

Mizrahi, T., and Abramson, J. (1985). Sources of strain between physicians and social workers: implications for social workers in health care settings, *Soc. Wk. in Hlth. Care*, **10**, 35–51.

Molony, C. H. (1975). Systematic valence coding of Mexican 'hot–cold' food, *Ecol. Food Nutr.*, **4**, 67–74.

Morley, D. (1980). The 'nationwide' audience, *British Film Institute*, London.

Morris, J. N., Chave, S. P., Adam, C., Sirey, C., and Epstein, L. (1973). Vigorous exercise in leisure time and the incidence of coronary heart disease, *Lancet*, i, 333–9.

Moser, K. A., Fox, A. J., and Jones, D. R. (1984). Unemployment and mortality in the OPCS Longitudinal Study, *Lancet*, ii, 1324–9.

MRFIT (Multiple Risk Factor Intervention Trial) Research Group (1982). The Multiple Risk Factor Intervention Trial–risk factor changes and mortality results. *J.A.M.A..*, **248**, 1465–76.

Murdoch, G. (1974). Mass communication and the construction of meaning, in *Reconstructing Social Psychology*, (ed. N. Armistead), Penguin, Harmondsworth, Middx, 205–20.

Murphy, J. F., Newcombe, R. G., and Sibert, J. R. (1982). The epidemiology of sudden infant death syndrome, *J. Epidem. Comm. Hlth*, **36**, 17–21.

Myrtek, M., and Villinger, U. (1976). Psychological and physiological effects of a 5-week ergometer training in healthy young men, *Med. Klin.*, **71**, 1623–30.

NACNE (National Advisory Council on Nutrition Education) (1983). *Proposals for Nutrition Guidelines for Health Education in Britain*, Health Education Council, London.

NCVO (National Council for Voluntary Organisations) (1979). *Directory of Community Health Initiatives*. London.

Naditch, M. P. (1984). The STAYWELL program in *Behavioural Health: A Handbook of Health Enhancement and Disease Prevention* (ed. J. D. Matarazzo, S. M. Weiss, J. A. Herd *et al.*), John Wiley & Sons, New York, 1071–1082.

Nathan, P. E. (1984). Johnson and Johnson's live for life: a comprehensive positive lifestyle change program, in *Behavioural Health: A Handbook of Health Enhancement and Disease Prevention* (ed. J. D. Matarazzo, S. M. Weiss, J. A. Herd *et al.*), John Wiley & Sons, New York, 1064–71.

National Board of Health and Welfare, Sweden (1985). *The Swedish Health Services in 1990's*, National Board of Health and Welfare Publications, Stockholm.

Navarro, V. (1975). The industrialisation of fetishism or the fetishism of industrialisation: a critique of Ivan Illich, *Int. J. Hlth Servs*, **5**, 351–71.

Navarro, V. (1976). Social class, political power and the state and their implications in medicine, *Soc. Sci. Med.*, **10**, 437–57.

Navarro, V. (1984). The crisis of the international capitalist order and its implications on the welfare state, in *Issues in the Political Economy of Health Care* (ed. J. B. McKinley), Tavistock, New York, 107–40.

Naylor, W. (1985). Walking time bombs, Aids and the press, *Med. Soc.*, **II**, 5–7.

Naytia, S. (1977). Social group and mortality in Finland, *B. J. Prev. Med.*, **31**, 231–6.

NCVO (National Council for Voluntary Organizations) (1979). *Directory of Community Health Initiatives*, NCVO, London.

Neilson, M. G. C., and Crofton, E. (1965). *The Social Effects of Chronic Bronchitis*, Chest and Heart Association, Edinburgh.

Neisser, U. (1976). *Cognition and Reality*, Freeman, San Francisco.

Neligman, G., Prudhma, D., and Steiner, H. (1974). *The Formative Years*, Oxford University Press and Nuffield Trust, London.

Newcomb, T. M., and Lessler, J. R. (1979). An expanded survey error model, in Panel on Incomplete Data of the Committee on National Statistics/National Research Council, *Symposium on Incomplete Data: Preliminary Proceedings*, US Department of Health, Education and Welfare, Social Security Administrative Office of Policy, Office of Research and Statistics, Washington DC.

Newman, J. P. (1984). Sex differences in symptoms of depression: clinical disorder or normal distress? *J. Hlth Soc. Behav.*, **25**, 136–59.

Newman, J. P. (1986). Gender, life strains, and depression, *J. Hlth Soc. Behav.*, **27**, 161–78.

Nichter, M. (1981). Idioms of distress: alternatives in the expression of psychosocial distress: a case study from South India, *Cult. Med. Psychiat.*, **5**, 379–408.

Nisbett, R. E. (1972). Hunger, obesity and the ventromedial hypothalmus, *Psychol. Rev.* **79**, 433–53.

Nixon, J., and Pearn, N. (1980). Norms for the social class distribution, *Med. J. Aust.*, **2**, 271–3.

Norman, R. M. (1986). *The Nature and Correlates of Health Behaviour*, Department of Health and Welfare, Ottawa, Canada.

OECD (Office for Economic Cooperation and Development) (1981). *The Welfare State in Crisis*, OECD Publications, Paris.

Office of Health Economics (1978). *Studies on Current Health Problems*, Nov. 63, *Birth Impairments*, Office of Health Economics, London.

Oliver, M. (1982). Does control of risk factors prevent coronary heart disease? *BMJ*, **285**, 1065–6.

OPCS (Office of Population Censuses and Surveys) Monitor (1978). *General Household Survey 1976*, HMSO, London.

OPCS (Office of Population Censuses and Surveys) Monitor (1985). *General Household Survey 1984*, HMSO, London.

Orbach, S. (1978). *Fat is a Feminist Issue*, Paddington, Hamlyn, London.

Oxford, J., and Edwards, G. (1977). *Alcoholism: A Comparison of Treatment and Advice with a Study of the Influence of Marriage*, Oxford University Press, Oxford.

Paffenbarger, R. S., and Hale, W. E. (1975). Work activity and coronary heart mortality, *New Eng. J. Med.*, **292**, 545–50.

Pamping, D. (1985). Evaluation in practice, in *Community Development in Health: Addressing the Issues* (ed. G. Somerville) King's Fund, London, 16–29.

Pamuk, E. R. (1985). Social class inequality in mortality from 1921 to 1972 in England and Wales, *Pop. Stud.*, **39**, 17–31.

Parkes, C. M. (1969). Broken heart: a statistical study of increased mortality among widows, *BMJ*, **1**, 744–746.

Parkes, C. M. (1979). The use of community care in prevention, in *New Methods of Mental Health Care* (ed. M. Meacher), Pergamon, Oxford, 49–68.

Parry, G. (1986). Paid employment, life events and social support and mental health in working class mothers, *J. Hlth Soc. Behav.*, 27, 193–208.

Parry, N. C. A., and Johnson, D. (1974). *Leisure and Social Structure*, final report to the Economic and Social Research Council, London.

Parsons, T. (1951). *The Social System*, Free Press of Glencoe, New York.

Pearse, I. H., and Crocker, L. H. (1943). *The Peckham Experiment*, Allen & Unwin, London.

Peck, C. (1982). *Controlling Chronic Pain*, Fontana, Sydney.

Pelletier, K. R. (1987). Database: research and evaluation results, *Am. J. Hlth Prom.*, 1, 66–8.

Pendleton, D. A. and Bochner, S. (1980). The communication of medical information in general practice consultations as a function of patient's social class, *Soc. Sci. Med.*, 14A, 669–73.

Phillips, M. R. (1984). The use of epidemiological models in planning preventive programmes in occupational health, in *System Science in Health Care* (eds. W. van Eimeren, R. Engelbrecht, and Ch. D. Flagle, Springer-Verlag, Berlin, 298–31.

Piaget, J. (1936). *La Naissance de l'intelligence chez l'enfant*, Delachaux et Niestle, Neuchâtel and Paris.

Piepe, A., Charlton, P., Morey, J., While, C., and Yerrell, P. (1986). Smoke opera? A content analysis of the presentation of smoking in TV soap, *Hlth Ed. J.*, 45, 199–203.

Pierret, J. (1986). What social groups think they can do about health; paper presented to World Health Organization Symposium on Health Behaviour: Its Application to Health Promotion, Pitlochry, to be published in *Behavioural Research in Health Promotion*, (provisional title) (eds. R. Anderson, J. K. Davies, I. Kickbush and D. V. McQueen), Oxford University Press, Oxford.

Pike, L. (1982). What are the links between housing and health? *Pulse*, 42, 5 June, 58.

Pike, M. C., Henderson, D. E., Drailo, M. D., Duke, A., and Roy, S. (1983). Breast cancer in young women and use of oral contraceptives: possible modifying effect of formulation and age at use, *Lancet*, 2, 926–30.

Pill, R. M. (1986). Health beliefs and health behaviour in local populations: the home environment; paper presented to World Health Organizations Symposium on Health Behaviour: Its Application in Health Promotion, Pitlochry, to be published in *Behavioural Research in Health Promotion* (provisional title) (eds. R. Anderson, J. K. Davies, I. Kickbush and D. V. McQueen), Oxford University Press, Oxford.

Pill, R. M., and Stott, N. C. H. (1982). Concepts of illness causation and responsibility: some preliminary data from a sample of working class mothers, *Soc. Sci. Med.*, 16, 43–52.

Pill, R. M. and Stott, N. C. H. (1985). Choice or change: further evidence on ideas of illness and responsibility for health, *Soc. Sci. Med.*, 20, 981–91.

Plant, M. (1985). *Women, Drinking and Pregnancy*, Tavistock, London.

Platt, S. D. (1987a). Unemployment and suicidal behaviour in Edinburgh, *Rad. Comm. Med.*, 30, 12–17.

Platt, S. D. (1987b). The aftermath of Angie's overdose: is soap (opera) damaging your health, *BMJ*, 294, 954–7.

Pochin, E. E. (1973). Levels of hazard in various occupations, in *The Assessment of Exposure and Risk* (ed. B. W. Duch), Society of Occupational Medicine, London, 33–58.

Polak, F. (1961). *The Image of Future*, Oceana, New York.

Popay, J., Griffiths, J., Draper, P., and Dennis, J. (1980). The impact of industrialisation on world health, in *Through the 80's: Thinking Global, Acting Locally* (ed. World Future Society), World Future Society Publications, Washington DC, 362–9.

Popham, R. E. (1970). Indirect methods of alcoholism prevalence estimation: a critical evaluation, in *Alcohol and Alcoholism* (ed. R. Popham), Toronto University Press, Toronto, 294–306.

Porter, T. M. (1986). *The Rise of Statistical Thinking: 1820–1900* Princeton University Press, Princeton, NJ.

Prochaska, J. O. and Di Clemente, C.E. (1982). Transtheoretical therapy: towards a more integrative model of change, *Psychotherapy: Theory, Research and Practice*, 19, 276–88.

Prochaska, J. O., and Di Clemente, C. E. (1983). Stages and processes of self-change of smoking: toward an integrative model of change', *J. Consult. Clin. Psychol.*, 51, 390–5.

Puska, P., Salonen, J., Nissinen, A., and Tuomilehto, J. (1983). Change in risk factors for coronary heart disease during ten years of a community intervention programme (North Karelia Project), *BMJ*, **287**, 1840.

Puska, P., Tuomilehto, J., Salonen, J., and Nissinen, A. (1981). *The North Karelia Project: Evaluation of a Comprehensive Community Program for the Control of Cardiovascular Diseases in 1972–77 in N Karelia, Finland*, World Health Organization, Copenhagen.

Raphael, B. (1977). Preventive intervention with the recently bereaved, *Arch. Gen. Psychiat.*, **34**, 1450–4.

Rappaport, R. N., Fogarty, M. P., and Rappaport, R. (eds), (1982). *Families in Britain*, Routledge & Kegan Paul, London.

Raw, M. (1977). The psychological modification of smoking, in *Contributions to Medical Psychology* (ed. S. Rachman), Pergamon, Oxford, 189–210.

Read, A. P., and Pease, K. (1971). How the press see the pill, *New Soc.*, **6 May**, 774–5.

Registrar-General (1978). *Occupational Mortality Tables 1970–72*, Decimal Supplement OPCS Series DS No. 1, HMSO, London.

Richman, N. (1976). Depression in mothers of pre-school children, *J. Child. Psychol. Psychiat.*, **17**, 75–8.

Rimpela, R. (1987). Heart disease and changing social conditions in Finland; paper presented at the Scotland 2000 Conference, Edinburgh.

Ringen, K. (1979). The new Fesnent in national health policy: the case of Norway's nutrition and food policy, *Soc. Sci. Med.*, **13C**, 33–41.

Ringen, K. (1983). Norway's nutrition and food policy: overview, results and future directions, in *Nutrition in the Community*, (2nd edn (ed. A. S. McLaren), John Wiley & Sons, New York, 159–69.

Rivers, W. H. R. (1924). *Medicine, Magic and Religion*, Harcourt Brace, New York.

Robbins, C. J. (ed.) (1978). *Food, Health and Farming*, Centre for Agricultural Strategy, CAS paper No. 7, University of Reading.

Roberts, H. (1985). *Patient Patients: Women and Their Doctors*, Pandora, Routledge & Kegan Paul, London.

Robertson, A. (1983). Managerialismo e pianificazione sanitaria: una critica alla riorganizzazione del Servizio Sanitario Britannico, in *Politiche di Welfare State e Modelli Decisionali* (eds. G. Bertin, M. Niero and E. Ziglio), Unicopli, Milan, 29–60.

Robertson, A. (1985). Trends in health policy: lessons from an international perspective, in *The Yearbook of Government in Scotland, 1985* (ed. D. McCrone), Unit for the Study of Government in Scotland, Edinburgh, 205–29.

Robertson, J. (1984). Scenarios for lifestyle and health, *Eur. Monog. Hlth Ed. Res.*, **6**, 151–72.

Robins, L., Davis, D., and Wish, E. (1977). Detecting predictors of rare events: demography of family and personality deviance as predictors of stages in the programme towards narcotics addiction, in *The Origins and Course of Psychopathology: Methods of Longitudinal Research* (eds. S. Strauss, H. Babigian and M. Roff), Plenum, New York, 241–52.

Rose, G., and Marmot, M. G. (1981). Social class and coronary heart disease, *B. Heart J.*, **45**, 13–19.

Rose, R. M. (1980). Endocrine response to stressful psychological events, *Psychiat. Clin. N. Am.*, **3**, 251–276.

Rosen, G. (1958). *A History of Public Health*, MD publications, New York.

Rosen, G. (1979). The evolution of social medicine, in *Handbook of Medical Sociology* (eds. H. E. Freeman, S. Levine and L. G. Reeder), Prentice-Hall, Englewood Cliffs, NJ, 23–70.

Rosenstock, I. M. (1966). Why people use health services, *Milb. Hem. Fd. Quart*, **44**, 54–127.

Rosenstock, I. M. (1974). Historical origins of the health belief model, *Hlth Ed. Monog.*, **2**, 328–35.

Roshier, B. (1976). The selection of crime news by the press, in *The Manufacture of News. Deviance, Social Problems and the Mass Media* (eds. S. Cohen and J. Young), Constable, London, 28–39.

Ross, C. E., and Huber, J. (1985). Hardship and depression, *J. Hlth Soc. Behav.*, **26**, 312–27.

Royal College of General Practitioners (1981). *What Sort of Doctor?* Report from General Practice No. 23, RCGP., London.

Royal College of Physicians (1977). *Smoking and Health*. Third Report, Pitman Medical Press, London.

Royal College of Physicians, (1980). *Medical Aspects of Dietary Fibre: Summary of a Report*, Pitman Medical Press, Tunbridge Wells.

Royal College of Physicians (1983). Obesity: a report, *J. Roy. Coll. Phys.*, **17**, 5–65.

Royal College of Psychiatrists (1986). *Alcohol: Our Favourite Drug*, Tavistock, London.

Royal College of Psychiatrists (1987). *A Great and Growing Evil*, Tavistock, London.

Royal Commission on the National Health Service (1979). *Report*. Cmnd. 7615 (Chairman, Sir Alex Morrison). HMSO, London.

Royal Norwegian Ministry of Agriculture (1975–6). On Norwegian nutrition and food policy; report No. 32 to the Storting, Oslo.

Royal Norwegian Ministry of Social Affairs (1981–2). On the follow-up of Norwegian nutrition policy; report No. 11 to the Storting, Oslo.

Rubin, D. B. (1978). Multiple imputations in sample surveys – a phenomenological Bayesian approach to nonresponse, in *Imputation and Editing of Faulty or Missing Survey Data* (eds. F. Aziz and F. Scheuren), US Department of Commerce, Bureau of the Census, Washington DC.

Rubin, D. B. (1979). *Handling Non-Response in Sample Surveys by Multiple Imputations*, monograph prepared for US Bureau of the Census, Washington DC.

Rush, D. (1981). Smoking, weight gain and nutrition during pregnancy, *Am. J. Obstet. Gynaec.*, **139**, 233–4.

Rush, D., and Cassano, P. (1983). Relationship of cigarette smoking and social class to birthweights and prenatal mortality among all births in Britain, 5–11 April 1970, *J. Epidem. Comm. Hlth*, **37**, 249–55.

Rutter, M., and Madge, J. (1976). *Cycles of Disadvantage*, Heinemann, London.

Ryle, J. A. (1940). Today and tomorrow, *BMJ*, **2**, 657.

Saltin, B., Nazar, K., Costill, D. L., Stein, E., Jansson, E., Essen, B., and Gollnick, P. D. (1976). The nature of the training response; peripheral and central adaptations to one-legged exercise, *Acta Physiol. Scand.*, **96**, 289–305.

Saunders, W., and Kershaw, P. (1979). Spontaneous remission from alcoholism: results from a community survey, B. J. Addict., **74**, 251–65.

Saunders, W., and Tate, D. (1983). Spontaneous remission revisited; paper presented at the 16th Scottish Alcohol Research Symposium, Pitlochry.

SCAN (*Scottish Community Action Newsletter*) (1987). April.

Schutz, A. (1970). *Reflections on the Problem of Relevance*, Yale University Press, New Haven, Conn.

Schutz, A. (1972). *The Phenomenology of the Social World*, Heinmann Educational Books, London.

Scottish Office (1984). *Community Care: Joint Planning and Support Finance*, NHS Circular No. 1985 (GEN) 18, Edinburgh.

Scott-Samuel, A. (1981). Social class inequality, access to primary care: a critique of recent research, *BMJ*, **283**, 510–11.

Selye, H. (1950), *The Physiology and Pathology of Exposure to Stress*, Acta, Montreal.

Seymour-Ure, C. (1968). *The Press Politics and the Public*, Methuen, London.

Shaper, A. G., Pock, S. J., Walker, M. Cohen, N. M., Wale, C. J. and Thomson, A. G. (1981). British Regional Heart Study: cardiovascular risk factors in middle aged men in 24 hours, *B. Med. J.*, **283**, 179–86.

Shaw, G. K., and Thomas, A. (1977). A joint psychiatric and medical outpatients' clinic for alcoholics, in *Alcoholism: New Knowledge and New Responses* (eds. G. Edwards and M. Grant), Croom Helm, London, 15–36.

Shaw, M. (1984). *Sport and Leisure Participation and Lifestyles in Different Residential Neighbourhoods: An Exploration of the ACORN Classification*, Sports Council/ESRC, London.

Shaw, M. (1986. Health promotion and the media: the soap opera, *Hlth Prom.*, **1**, 211–12.

Sherlock, S. (1982). Alcohol and disease, *B. Med. Bull*, Churchill Livingstone, London, **38**, 67–70.

SHHD (Scottish Home and Health Department) (1977). *The Health Service in Scotland: The Way Ahead*, HMSO, Edinburgh.

Sidney, K. H., Shephard, R. J., and Harrison, J. E. (1977). Endurance training and body composition of the elderly, *Am. J. Clin. Nutr.*, **30**, 326–33.

Simpson, W. J. (1957). A preliminary report on cigarette smoking and the incidence of prematurity, *Am. J. Obstet. Gynaecol.*, **73**, 808–15.

Skinner, B. F. (1948). *Walden Two*, Macmillan, New York.

Skrabanek, P. (1985). False premises and false promises of breast cancer screening. *Lancet*, **August 10th**, 316–18.

Skrimshire, A. (1978). *Area Disadvantage, Social Class and the Health Service*, Social Evaluation Unit, University of Glasgow.

Slater, C. H, Lorimor, R. J., and Lairson, D. R. (1985). The independent contributions of socioeconomic status and health practices to health status, *Prev. Med.*, **14**, 372–8.

Smith, A. (1974). *The British Press since the War*, David & Charles, Newton Abbot.

Social Democratic Party (1982). *Fair Treatment: Social Democracy in the Health and Social Services*, SDP Policy Department, London.

Sommerville, G. (1984). *Community Development in Health: Addressing the Confusions*, King's Fund Centre, London.

Sorensen, A. B. (1986). Progress in studying change, *Am. J. Sociol.*, **92**, 691–6.

South Manchester Health Authority (1982). *An Evaluation of Manchester Well Woman Clinic*, SMHA., Manchester

Spencer, B. (1987). The South Manchester Family Worker Scheme, *Hlth Prom.* **2**, 29–38.

Stacey, M. (1986). Concepts of health and illness and the division of labour in health care, in *Concepts of Health. Illness and Disease* (eds. C. Currer and M. Stacey). Berg Publications, Leamington Spa, Hamburg and New York. 9–27.

Stein, H. (1985). *The Psychodynamics of Medical Practice*, University of California Press, Berkeley, Calif.

Stephens, B., Mason, J. P., and Isely, R. B. (1985). Health and low-cost housing, *World Hlth For.*, **6**, 59–62.

Stephens, T., Jacobs, D., and White, C. (1985). A descriptive epidemiology of leisure time physical activity, *Pub. Hlth*, **100**, 147–58.

Sterling, P., and Eyer, J. (1981). Biological basis of stress-related mortality. *Soc. Sci. Med.*, **15E**, 3–42.

Sterling, T. D. (1978). Does smoking kill workers or does working kill smokers? or the relationship between smoking, occupation and respiratory disease. *Int. J. Hlth Servs.*, **8**, 437–52.

Stern, J. (1983). Social mobility and the interpretation of social class mortality differentials, *J. Soc. Pol.*, **12**, 27–49.

Sternbach, R. A., and Tursky, B. (1965). Ethnic differences among housewives in psychophysical and skin potential responses to electric shock, *Psychophysiol.*, **1**, 241–6.

Stimson, G. V., and Webb, B. (1975). *Going to See the Doctor: The Consultation Process in General Practice*, Routlege & Kegan Paul, London.

Stoller, E. P. (1984). Self-assessments of health by the elderly: the impact of informal assistance, *J. Hlth Soc. Behav.*, **25**, 260–70.

Strachan, D., and Elton, R. (1986). Respiratory morbidity in children and the home environment, *Fam. Pract.*, **92**, 137–42.

Strauss, R. A. (1981). The theoretical frame of symbolic interactionism: a contextualist social science, *Symb. Interact.*, **4**, 261–81.

Strom, T. B., and Carpenter, C. B. (1980). Cyclic nucleotides in immunosuppression: neuroendocrine pharmacologic manipulation and in vivo regulation of immunity acting via second messenger systems, *Transpl. Proc.*, **12**, 304–10.

Sudnow, D. (1967). *Passing On: The Social Organisation of Dying*, Prentice-Hall, Englewood Cliffs, N.J.

Susman, G. I., and Evered, R. D. (1978). An assessment of the scientific merits of action research, *Admin. Sci. Quart.*, **23**, 582–603.

Sykes, W., and Hoinville, G. (1985). *Telephone Interviewing on a Survey of Social Attitudes: A Comparison with Face-to-Face Procedures*, Survey Research Centre Publication, London.

Syme, S. L. (1976). *Hypertension Education Program in a Low Income Community*, final report on

NIH grant No. HL16959 (National High Blood Pressure Education Program), Washington DC.

Syme, S. L. (1986). Strategies for health promotion, *Prev. Med.*, **15**, 492–507.

Syme, S. L., and Berkman, Lisa, F. (1976). Social class, susceptibility and sickness, *Am. J. Epidem*, **104**, 1–13.

Tannahill, A. (1985). What is health promotion? *Hlth Ed. J.*, **44**, 167–8.

Tannenbaum, P. H. (1953). Effects of headlines on the interpretation of news stories, *J. Quart.*, **30**, 189–97.

Tanur, J. M. (1983). Methods for large-scale surveys and experiments, in *Sociological Methodology 1983–4* (ed. S. Leinhardt), Jossey-Bass, San Francisco, 1–79.

Taussig, M. T. (1980). Reification and the consciousness of the patient, *Soc. Sci. Med.*, **14B**, 3–13.

Taylor, R., and Ford, G. (1981). Lifestyle and aging: three traditions in lifestyle research, *Aging and Society*, **1**, 329–45.

Teitelbaum, J. M. (1969). Lamta: leadership and social organisation of a Tunisian community, unpublished PhD thesis, University of Manchester.

Tennant, C., and Andrews, G. (1987). The pathogenic quality of life event stress in neurotic impairment, *Arch. Gen. Psychiat.*, **35**, 859–63.

Tennant, C., and Bebbington, P. (1978). The social causation of depression: a critique of Brown and his colleagues, *Psychol. Med.*, **8**, 1–11.

Theorell, T., Lind, E., and Floderus, G. (1975). The relationship of disturbing life-changes to the early development of myocardial infarction and other serious illnesses, *Int. J. Epidem.*, **3**, 281–7.

Thoits, P. A. (1982). Conceptional, methodological and theoretical problems in studying social support and a buffer against life stress, *H. Hlth Soc. Behav.*, **23**, 145–59.

Thomas, D. (1983). *The Making of Community Work*, Allen & Unwin, London.

Tibblin, G., Wilhelmsen, L., and Werko, L. (1975). Risk factors for myocardial infarction and death due to ischemic heart disease and other causes, *Am. J. Cardiol.*, **35**, 514–22.

Tilson, H. H. (1984). Governmental legislative policies to control and direct the promotion of health, in *Oxford Textbook of Public Health, volume 1* (eds. W. W. Holland, R. Detels and G. Knox), Oxford University Press, Oxford, 161–9.

Timio, M., Gentili, S., and Pede, S. (1979). Free adrenaline and noradrenaline excretion related to occupation stress, *B. Heart. J.*, **42**, 471–4.

Tinbergen, N. (1951). *The Study of Instinct*, Oxford University Press, Oxford.

Titmuss, R. M. (1968). *Commitment to Welfare*, Allen & Unwin, London.

Townsend, P. (1979). *Poverty in the United Kingdom*, Penguin, Harmondsworth, Middx.

Townsend, P., and Davidson, N. (1982). *Inequalities in Health: The Black Report*, Penguin, Harmondsworth, Middx.

Trist, E. (1979). New directions of hope: recent innovations interconnecting organisational, industrial, community and personal development, *Refer. Stud.*, **13**, 439–51.

Tsalikis, G. (1980). Remodelling the staff of Aescalapius, *Soc. Sci. Med.*, **14A**, 97–106.

Tsalikis, G. (1984). The consequences of Canadian health policies, in *Issues in Canadian Social Policy*, Volume 2, Canadian Council of Social Development, Ottawa, 121–60.

Tuchfeld, B. (1981). Spontaneous remission in alcoholics: empirical observations and theoretical implications, *J. Stud. Alc.*, **42**, 624–41.

Tudor-Hart, J. (1971). The inverse care law, *Lancet*, **i**, 7696.

Tuma, N. B., and Hannan, M. T. (1984). *Social Dynamics: Models and Methods*, Academic Press, Orlando, Florida.

Tupek, A. R. and Richardson, W. J. (1978). Use of ratio estimates to compensate for non-response bias in certain economic surveys, in *Imputation and Editing of Faulty or Missing Survey Data* (eds. F. F. Aziz and F. Scheuren), US Department of Commerce, Bureau of the Census, Washington DC.

Turner, C. F., and Martin, E. (eds.) (1984). *Surveying Subjective Phenomena*, Volume 1, Russell Sage Foundation, New York.

Turpeinen, O., Karvonen, M. K., Pekkarinen, M., Miettinen, M., Eluoso, R., and Paavilainen,

E. (1979). Dietary prevention of coronary heart disease: the Finnish Mental Hospital Study, *Int. J. Epidem.*, **8**, 99–118.

Turton, P. (1983). Medicine and the media, *BMJ*, **286**, 554.

Unschuld, P. U. (1986). The conceptualsation (Überformung) of individual and collective experiences of illness, in *Concepts of Health, Illness and Disease* (eds. C. Currer and M. Stacey), Berg Publications, Leamington Spa, Hamburg and New York, 51–70.

Urquhart, J. (1987). The assessment of leukaemia data by the Dounreay Planning Inquiry, *Rad. Comm. Med.*, **Autumn**, 20–7.

USDHEW (United States Department of Health Education and Welfare) (1979). *Smoking and Health: A Report of the Surgeon-General*, DHEW Publn Nc. (PHS) 79–50066, US Government Printing Office, Washington DC.

USDHEW (United States Department of Health Education and Welfare) (1979). *Healthy People: The Surgeon-General's Report on Health Provision and Disease Prevention*, US Government Printing Office, Washington DC.

USHP (Unit for the Study of Health Policy) (1978). *The NHS in the Next 30 Years: A New Perspective on the Health of the British*, Guy's Hospital Medical School, USHP, Department of Community Medicine, London.

Uutela, A. (1986). Perceived health consequences of smoking, assumed difficulty of quitting, and intentions to quit smoking; paper presented at the 21st International Congress of Applied Psychology, 13–18 July, Jerusalem.

Valaskakis, K. (1981). The conserver society: emerging paradigm of the 1980s? *Futurist*, **April**, 5–13.

Valaskakis, K., Sindell, P. S., Smith G., and Fitzpatrick-Martin, I. (1979). *The Conserver Society: A Workable Alternative for the Future*, Harper & Row, New York.

Valliant, G. (1983). *The Natural History of Alcoholism*, Harvard University Press, Cambridge, Mass.

Van den Heuvel, W. J. A. (1978). Participants and non-participants in a mammography mass screening: who is who? in *Breast Cancer* (eds. P. C. Brand and P. A. Keep), MTP Press, London, 91–6.

Van Loon, R. J. (1980). From shared cost to block funding and beyond: the policies of health insurance in Canada in *Perspectives on Canadian Health Policy: History and Emerging Trusts* (eds. C. A. Meilicke and J. L. Storch), Health Administration Press, Ann Arbor, Mich., 342–66.

Varheit, G., Holzer, C., and Schwab, J. (1973). An analysis of social class and racial differences in depressive symptom – aetiology: a community study, *J. Hlth Soc. Behav.*, **4**, 921–99.

Vartiainen, E., Puska, P., Koskela, K., Nissinen, A., and Toumilehto, J. (1986). Ten year results of a community-based anti-smoking program (as part of the North Karelia project in Finland), *Hlth Ed. Res.*, **1**, 175–84.

Vaughn, C. E., and Leff. J. P. (1976). The influence of family and social factors on the course of psychiatric illness: a comparison of schizophrenic and depressed neurotic patients, *B.J. Psychiat.*, **129**, 125–37.

Verbrugge, L. M. (1985). Gender and health: an up-date on hypothesis and evidence, *J. Hlth Soc. Behav.*, **26**, 156–82.

Vessey, M. P., Lawless, M., McPherson, K., and Yeates, D. (1983). Neoplasia of the cervix uteri and contraception: a possible adverse effect of the pill, *Lancet*, **ii**, 930–4.

Wadsworth, J. Burnell, I., Taylor, B., and Butler, N. (1983). Family type and accidents in pre-school children, *J. Epidem. Comm. Hlth*, **37**, 100–4.

Wadsworth, M. E. J., Butterfield, W., and Blaney, H. (1973). *Health and Illness: The Choice of Treatment*, Tavistock, London.

Waerness, K. (1978). The invisible welfare state: women's work at home, *Acta Sociol.*, **Suppl.**, 193–207.

Wagner, R. V. (1969). The study of attitude change: an introduction, in *The Study of Attitude Change* (eds. R. V. Wagner and J. J. Sherwood), Brooks-Cole, Belmont, Calif., 1–18.

Waitzkin, H. (1985). Information giving in medical care, *J. Hlth Soc. Behav.*, **26**, 81–101.

Warheit, C. J. (1979). Life events, coping, stress and depression. *Am. J. Psychiat.*, **136**, 502–5.

Warner, H. L. (1977). Health hazard appraisal, an instrument for change, *Proceedings of the 13th Meeting of the Society of Prospective Medicine*, 120–3.

Warr, P. B. (1984). Job loss, unemployment and pyschological well-being, in *Role Transitions* (eds. V. L. Allen and E. van de Vliert). Plenum, London, p. 31–45.

Warr, P. B., and Parry, G. (1982). Paid employment and women's psychological well-being, *Psychol. Bull.*, **91**, 498–516.

Warr, P. B., and Payne, R. L. (1982). Experiences of strain and pleasure among British adults, *Soc. Sci. Med.*, **16**, 1691–7.

Weaver, Sir L. (1926). *Cottages*, London.

Wedge, P., and Prosser, H. (1973). *Born to Fail?* Arrow Books, London.

Weinblatt, E., Shapiro, S., and Frank, C. W. (1971). Changes in personal characteristics of men, over five years, following first diagnosis of coronary heart disease, *Am. J. Pub. Hlth*, **61**, 831–7.

Weiner, C. (1980). *The Politics of Alcoholism*, The Transaction Press, NJ.

Weiss, C. H. (ed.) (1977). *Using Social Research in Policy Making*, Heath, D. C. Heath, Lexington, Mass.

Weiss, C. H., Kosse, G., Wagenaar, H., Kliprogge, J., and Vorbeck, M. (1982). Policy research in the context of diffuse decision-making, in *Social Science Research and Public Policy Making: A Reappraisal*, NFER. Windsor, England, 288–314.

Weller, G. R., and Manga, P. (1983). The development of health policy in Canada, in *The Politics of Canadian Public Policy* (eds. M. M. Atkinson and M. A. Chandler), University of Toronto Press, Toronto, 223–46.

Wellin, E. (1955). Water boiling in a Peruvian town, in *Health, Culture and Community: Case Studies of Public Reactions to Health Programmes* (ed. B. D. Paul), Russell Sage Foundation, New York, 71–106.

Wellin, E. (1958). Implications of local culture for public health, *Hum. Org.*, **16**, 16–18.

Wellings, K. (1985). Help or hype: an analysis of media coverage of the 1983 'pill scare', in *Health Education and the Media Preprints of 2nd International Conference, Edinburgh* (eds. D. S. Leather, G. B. Hastings, K. M. O'Reilly and J. K. Davies), Pergamon, London, 109–15.

Wenzel, E. (1983). Lifestyles and living conditions and their impact on health: a report of the meeting, in *Lifestyles and Health: European Monographs in Health Education Research*, World Health Organization, Scottish Health Education Group, 1–50.

West, P. B. (1979). Making sense of epilepsy, in *Social Aspects, Attitudes, Communication, Care and Training* (eds. D. J. Osborne, M. M. Grunberg and J. R. Eiser), Academic Press, London, 35–48.

West, R. R., and Lowe, C. R. (1976). Mortality from ischaemic heart disease: inter-town variation and its association with climate in England and Wales, *Int. J. Epidem.*, **5**, 195–9.

Westman, M., Eden, D., and Shirom, A. (1985). Job stress, cigarette smoking and cessation: the conditioning effects of peer support, *Soc. Sci. Med.*, **20**, 637–44.

Whitehead, M. (1987). *The Health Divide*, Health Education Council, London.

WHO (World Health Organization) (1948). Official Records of the World Health Organization, No. 2, UNWHO, Interim Commission, Geneva, 100.

WHO (World Health Organization) (1975). Report on the Director-General, WHO, Geneva.

WHO (World Health Organization) (1978). Primary Health Care; report of the International Conference on Primary Health Care, Alma-Ata, September, Geneva.

WHO (World Health Organization) (1982). Lifestyles and their impact on health, Technical Discussion Paper, EUR/RC33/Tech.Disc. 1, WHO (Euro), Copenhagen.

WHO (World Health Organization) (1983). Primary prevention of essential hypertension: Report of a WHO meeting, Geneva.

WHO (World Health Organization) (1984). *Health Promotion: A Discussion Document on the Concept and Principles*, WHO (Euro), Health Education Unit Publications, Copenhagen.

WHO (World Health Organization) (1985). *Targets for Health for All*, WHO (Euro), Copenhagen.

WHO (World Health Organization) (1986a). Ottawa Charter for Health Promotion, *J. Hlth Prom.*, **1**, i–v.

WHO (World Health Organization) (1986b). *Framework for a Health Promotion Policy: A Discussion Document*, WHO (Euro), Copenhagen.

WHO (World Health Organization) (1986c). *International Action for Health: The Role of Intersectoral Cooperation in National Strategies for Health for All*, WHO, Geneva.

WHO (World Health Organization) (1987). *Health Policy and Health Promotion: Towards a New*

Concept of Public Health, report on a WHO meeting, Baden, Vienna, 6–11 September 1986, WHO (Euro), Copenhagen.

Wicker, A. W. (1971). An examination of the 'other variables' explanation of attitude behaviour inconsistency, *J. Pers. Soc. Psychol.*, **19**, 18–25.

Wildavsky, A. (1977). Doing better and feeling worse: the political pathology of health policy, in *Doing Better and Feeling Worse* (ed. J. Knowles), Health in the United States, Daedalus, NY, 105–23.

Wiley, J. A., and Comacho, T. C. (1980). Life-style and future health: evidence from the Alameda County Study, *Prev. Med.*, **9**, 1–21.

Wilkinson, R. G. (1986). Socio-economic differences in mortality, in *Class and Health: Research and Longitudinal Data* (ed. R. G. Wilkinson), Tavistock, London, 1–20.

Wille, R. (1978). Preliminary communication: cessation of opiate dependency: procedures involved in achieving abstinence, *B. J. Add.*, **73**, 381–4.

Wille, R. (1980). Processes of recovery among heroin users, in *Drug Problems in the Sociocultural Context*, Public Health Paper No. 73, World Health Organization, Geneva.

Williams, R. (1983). Concepts of health: an analysis of lay logic, *Sociol.*, **17**, 185–205.

Williams, R. W. (1966). *Communications*, rev. edn, Chatto, London.

Wilner, D. M. Robbins, S., and Bernard, T. (1962). *The housing environment and family life. A longitudinal study of the effects of housing on morbidity and mental health*, Johns Hopkins Medical School, Baltimore.

Windsor, R. A., Baranowski, T., Clark, N., and Cutter, G. (1984). *Evaluation of Health Promotion and Education Programs*, Mayfield Publishing, Palo Alto, Calif.

Wing, J. K., and Hailey, A. M. (eds.) (1972). *Evaluating a Community Psychiatric Service*, Oxford University Press, London.

Winnick, C. (1962). Maturing out of Narcotics addiction, *Bull. Narc.*, **14**, 1–9.

Winship, C., and Mare, R. D. (1983). Structural equations and path analysis for discrete data, *Am. J. Sociol.*, **89**, 54–110.

Wiseman, C. (1978). Selections of major planning issues, *Pol. Sci.*, **9**, 71–86.

Wiseman, C. (1979). Strategic planning in the Scottish health service: a mixed-scanning approach, *Long Range Planning*, **12**, 103–13.

Witschi, J., Singer, M., Wu-Lee, M., and Stare, F. (1978). Family cooperation and effectiveness in a cholesterol lowering diet, *J. Am. Diet Ass.*, **72**, 384–9.

Wooff, K., Freeman, H. L., and Fryers, T. (1983). Psychiatric service use in Salford, *B. J. Psychiat.*, **142**, 588–97.

Wright, S. (1934). The method of path coefficients, *Anns of Math. Stats*, **5**, 161–215.

Wrightsman, L. S. (1966). Wallace supporters and adherence to 'law and order', *J. Pers. Soc. Psychol.*, **4**, 328–33.

Yarrow, A. (1986), *Politics, Society, and Preventive Medicine*, Nuffield Provincial Hospital Trust, Occasional Papers 6, London.

Young, A. (1976). Some implications of medical beliefs and practices for social anthropology, *Am. Anthrop.*, **78**, 5–24.

Young, A. (1982). The anthropologies of illness and sickness, *Ann. Rev. Anthrop.*, **11**, 257–85.

Zborowski, M. (1952). Cultural components in response to pain, *J. Soc. Issues*, **8**, 16–30.

Ziesat, H. A. (1977). Behaviour modification in the treatment of hypertension, *Int. J. Psychiat. Med.*, **8**, 257–63.

Ziglio, E. (1983). Considerazioni metodologiche per la formulazione delle politiche di health promotion, in *Politiche de welfare state e modelli decisionali* (eds. G. Bertin, M. Niero and E. Ziglio), Unicopli, Milan, 311–19.

Ziglio, E. (1985). Uncertainty and innovation in health policy: the Canadian and Norwegian approaches to health promotion, *PhD thesis*, Department of Social Administration, University of Edinburgh.

Ziglio, E. (1986). Uncertainty and innovation in health promotion: nutrition policy in two countries, *Hlth Prom.*, **1**, 257–69.

Ziglio, E. (1987a). A new perspective on health policy: analysis of the Lalonde Report a decade after its publication, University of Edinburgh, Research Unit in Health and Behavioural Change Working Paper No. 16.

Ziglio, E. (1987b). Uncertainties and dilemmas in future health policy scenarios: some cautionary issues, *Fut. Res. Quart.*, Forthcoming publication.

Ziglio, E. (1987c). Policy-making in conditions of uncertainty: the case of health promotion policy, University of Edinburgh, Research Unit in Health and Behavioural Change Working Paper No. 7.

Zimbardo, P. G. (1970). The human choice: individuation, reason and order versus deindividuation, impulse and chaos, in *Nebraska Symposium on Motivation* (eds. W. J. Arnold and D. Levine), University of Nebraska Press, Lincoln, Nebr. 237–307.

Zola, I. (1975). In the name of health and illness, *Soc. Sci. Med.*, **9**, 83–7.

Zola, I. K. (1973). Pathways to the doctor. from person to patient, *Soc. Sci. Med.*, **7**, 677–89.

Index